THE
HEALTHY HOME
COOKBOOK

Diabetes-Friendly Recipes for Holidays, Parties, and Everyday Celebration

BARBARA SEELIG-BROWN

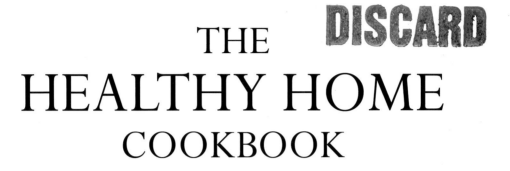

American Diabetes Association.

Director, Book Publishing, Abe Ogden; Managing Editor, Greg Guthrie; Acquisitions Editor, Victor Van Beuren; Editor, Rebekah Renshaw; Production Manager, Melissa Sprott; Composition, pixiedesign, llc; Cover Design, Vis-á-Vis Creative Concepts; Photographer, Renee Comet; Printer, R.R. Donnelley.

Printed in the United States of America
1 3 5 7 9 10 8 6 4 2

The suggestions and information contained in this publication are generally consistent with the Clinical Practice Recommendations and other policies of the American Diabetes Association, but they do not represent the policy or position of the Association or any of its boards or committees. Reasonable steps have been taken to ensure the accuracy of the information presented. However, the American Diabetes Association cannot ensure the safety or efficacy of any product or service described in this publication. Individuals are advised to consult a physician or other appropriate health care professional before undertaking any diet or exercise program or taking any medication referred to in this publication. Professionals must use and apply their own professional judgment, experience, and training and should not rely solely on the information contained in this publication before prescribing any diet, exercise, or medication. The American Diabetes Association—its officers, directors, employees, volunteers, and members—assumes no responsibility or liability for personal or other injury, loss, or damage that may result from the suggestions or information in this publication.

♾ The paper in this publication meets the requirements of the ANSI Standard Z39.48-1992 (permanence of paper).
ADA titles may be purchased for business or promotional use or for special sales. To purchase more than 50 copies of this book at a discount, or for custom editions of this book with your logo, contact the American Diabetes Association at the address below, at booksales@diabetes.org, or by calling 703-299-2046.

American Diabetes Association
1701 North Beauregard Street
Alexandria, Virginia 22311

DOI: 10.2337/9781580405157

Library of Congress Cataloging-in-Publication Data
Seelig-Brown, Barbara.
  The healthy home cookbook : diabetes-friendly recipes for holidays, parties, and everyday celebrations / Barbara Seelig-Brown.
       pages cm
  Summary: "Whether it's a holiday celebration, an after-church family get-together, or just a small dinner party among friends, food is central to almost any gathering of family and friends. Designed around the notion that everyone should enjoy hearty family favorites or adventurous party bites, Barbara Seelig-Brown has pulled together a collection of healthy dishes and festive recipes that everyone in a group can enjoy. Each recipe is designed to be flavorful and satisfying yet healthy. The days of separate foods for partygoers are a thing of the past. Now anyone looking to entertain can feature a full spread with dishes that everyone can enjoy guilt-free. From small bites to get-togethers, full courses for a dinner party, to satisfying favorites for a Sunday football marathon, The Healthy Home Cookbook is packed with recipes and meal-planning tips that will have everyone wanting more"-- Provided by publisher.
  Includes bibliographical references and index.
  ISBN 978-1-58040-515-7 (pbk.)
  1. Diabetes--Diet therapy--Recipes. 2. Diabetics--Nutrition. 3. Holiday cooking. 4. Parties. I. Title.
RC662.S446 2013
641.5'6314--dc23
                      2013022196

Contents

Dedication and Acknowledgments

For Adam and Dave: with love, gratitude, and appreciation for you and all that you have given me, including your wonderful families.

Acknowledgments

Thank you to my friends and family who consistently serve as my recipe testers. You are all full of great ideas and have allowed me the joy of cooking for you. To my dream friends, Laurie and Val Burzynski, many thanks for sharing your favorite Italian family recipes. To Barone: without whose support I would not have been on this journey. Thanks to my sister, brother, and their families for their support, especially the last few years. And thanks to my mom and dad for the wonderful family table we always enjoyed.

To the staff at the American Diabetes Association: Rebekah Renshaw, for her generous editing and patience; Abe Ogden for considering the idea for this book; and to Carrie Engle and Heschel Falek for marketing The Diabetes Seafood Cookbook *and* The Stress Free Diabetes Kitchen *in a way that made this book possible. Additional thanks to Renee Comet, Lisa Cherkasky, and Carolyn Schimley for the beautiful photography and food styling, and to pixiedesign, llc, for the beautiful design of this book.*

Thank you all with love and appreciation.

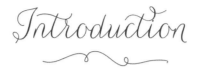

Introduction

I love to have family and friends at my table. I love to entertain! But I think that "entertaining" can be a scary word for many and we don't want anyone to feel overwhelmed, so I present this book to you. Cooking for friends and family is a gift. When you spend time in the kitchen you show your love for those whom you are cooking for.

People eat out or get takeout so frequently these days that entertaining at home is truly a treat. Visits with friends and family are more relaxed and more meaningful when you're at home. We are currently seeing a marked trend in a return to cooking at home. Our kitchens are now the new living rooms, making entertaining more casual and less daunting. I try to make my home welcoming by creating a "help yourself" atmosphere. You can set up areas of your kitchen, family room, living room, dining room, or any space that are inviting with simple touches like glasses near the wine bar or coffee cups near the coffee maker. I want my guests to be comfortable and relaxed, so as a hostess, I also need to be relaxed. While there are books that have been published on entertaining, they do not always include recipes that meet the American Diabetes Association standards. Make your experience be a healthy one!

My mission is to get the home cook to realize that cooking is an essential part of a healthy lifestyle and can offer the added bonus of being more economical. When you cook, you are more in control of your food intake. Why not take this beyond your everyday meals into entertaining as well? You can eat better-quality food because it is more economical than prepared food. I provide a healthy pantry list as well as quick, delicious recipes that focus on the importance of fresh, quality ingredients. If you use quality ingredients, you have to do less to the dish and you save time. Also, cooking at home is more enjoyable than standing in a takeout line. I would much rather be relaxed at home in my bunny slippers, cooking for my family, than fighting the crowds at the takeout window. I encourage people to think of cooking as a pleasant experience. Relax, keep a well-stocked pantry (page vii), and use my delicious, quick, and easy recipes that focus on quality of ingredients rather than lots of ingredients.

How to Read a Recipe

Are you sometimes confused or intimidated by the way a recipe is written? Do things come out differently than you expected? As a professional recipe developer, I follow certain guidelines, the gold standards, if you will, for writing recipes. My goal is to make my recipes as clear as possible so that you will enjoy cooking at home and do it more often.

One very important point that I like to bring up to my readers and students is that there are many variables in a recipe. Variables can be things like interpretation, pan size, type of pan, type of stove, ingredient quality, atmosphere, and so much more. If a recipe does not turn out perfectly, it is not necessarily your fault. It could be the result of one of the variables. Since our stoves, equipment, and ingredient quality can vary greatly, recipes should include descriptors such as: Cook chicken breast 3 minutes on each side or **until golden brown on each side**. Perhaps the recipe developer had a gas stove and yours is electric. The timing will vary greatly but the end result can still be similar by noting the descriptor—*golden brown.* Is the quality of the recipe developer's pan and your pan identical? It is highly unlikely that we all have the same supplies and equipment in our kitchens.

Ingredients should be listed in the order in which they are added in the preparation or cooking method. Terms should be basic when there are multiple words available. For example, not everyone knows how to braise but they are likely to understand the term simmer.

Mise en place is your best friend! This means that you read the recipe thoroughly and perform all necessary prep before turning on the stove, mixer, or food processor. If the recipe prep calls for pounded chicken or sliced mushrooms, do it as part of the *mise en place*. Measure the stock, peel the garlic, chop the onions, and zest the lemon. Does the recipe call for ingredients at room temperature? This can take 20–30 minutes once removed from the refrigerator. Does something need to be defrosted? *Mise en place* will help guide you through the cooking process. For instance, sautéing garlic takes only minutes but pounding the chicken breast can take much longer. The pounding should be done before the garlic hits the pan to avoid scorching the garlic.

USER GUIDELINES

- Always read a recipe in its entirety before starting the cooking process
- Be sure that you have all ingredients on hand
- Be sure that you understand all the techniques and terms in the recipe
- Prepare a *Mise en Place*
- Look for descriptors
- Trust your judgment
- Don't be intimidated
- Have fun

Healthy Pantry List

Keeping the house well stocked allows more time for cooking. Why make multiple trips to the grocery store when you can keep so many staple items on hand at all times. I would rather be home in my bunny slippers, listening to my favorite CD, and sipping wine while preparing dinner for my family, than standing in a take out or grocery store line.

PANTRY

- Extra virgin olive oil
- Balsamic, white balsamic, and wine vinegars
- Sea salt—fine grind
- Garlic—fresh, whole heads
- Onions
- Shallots
- Whole pepper and a good-quality pepper mill
- All-purpose flour
- Yeast
- Honey
- Sugar blends
- Pasta—a variety of shapes and sizes
- Rice—jasmine, arborio
- Beans—canned, a variety to include: black beans, pink beans, chickpeas, small white beans
- Lentils—DePuy, brown, and red
- Polenta/corn meal
- Evaporated skim milk
- Canned broth and stock—low-sodium chicken, beef, mushroom, vegetable
- Diced tomatoes, crushed tomatoes, and tomato paste
- Anchovies—rolled fillets with capers
- Clams
- Fruits—dried such as raisins, cherries, and apricots
- Fruits—canned such as mandarin oranges, apricots, crushed pineapple
- Salt & Pepper Blend (see page viii)

REFRIGERATOR

- Low-fat cottage cheese
- Part-skim and no-fat ricotta
- Crumbled gorgonzola
- Low-fat plain yogurt
- Light cream cheese bricks, also labeled Neufchatel (1/3 less fat)
- Fresh mozzarella
- Parmigiano-Reggiano cheese
- Eggs—large
- Mustard—variety
- Capers
- Vermouth—dry white
- Wine—dry white
- Lemons, Limes, Oranges
- Salad greens—a variety of types, textures, and colors
- Fresh baby spinach
- Carrots
- Celery
- Fresh herbs—basil, oregano, rosemary
- Sun-dried tomatoes—not in oil
- Olives

FREEZER

- Filled pastas—such as tortellini and agnolotti
- Homemade breadcrumbs
- Artichokes
- Baby corn
- Peas
- String beans—whole
- Pearl onions
- Ground beef and/or buffalo
- Turkey cuts—such as ground, breast, sausage
- Chicken breast—boneless and skinless, individually wrapped
- Roasting chickens—5–6 pounds, washed and then frozen
- Large shrimp, cooked, peeled and deveined
- Large shrimp, uncooked, peeled and deveined
- Individually frozen fish fillets, such as whiting or halibut
- Individually frozen center-cut pork chops

- Blueberries, raspberries, strawberries
- Pignoli (pine nuts)
- Crepes

ADDITIONAL ITEMS

- Anything you love to cook with!

Many of us keep a bowl of fine sea salt on the counter for seasoning. A pinch is about 1/8 of a teaspoon. Another quick shortcut is to make my stress free **Salt & Pepper Blend** by mixing 2 parts fine sea salt with 1 part ground black pepper. Keep it handy on the counter for quick seasoning of the recipes in this book. You will see references to it throughout this book.

By keeping these items on hand, you will be able to come home from a busy day and put together a colorful, delicious meal in no time using the recipes found in any of my cookbooks.

Basic Wine Pairing

There are many food and wine pairing philosophies. It is likely that you already have your own favorite foods. When you begin trying different wines, you will also discover favorites. Wine should not be a mystery. They should be enjoyed and thought of as something of interest and pleasure. Once you are comfortable with your own pairings, you can walk into a reputable wine store armed with your favorite recipes, ask for help, and turn a great meal into something wonderful.

PAIRING TIPS

Drink what you like with the food that you like. While this may sound oversimplified, it speaks to the fact that there is so much out there to choose from. So why not? Perhaps your taste leans toward spicy food. It is likely that you will also lean toward a fuller bodied wine with spicy notes.

One of my personal favorite guidelines for pairing is to keep the wines local. So, drink Italian wine with Italian dishes and Portuguese wine with Portuguese food. Along the same lines, I also pair casual wine with casual food and Champagne with hors d'oeuvres and special-occasion foods. Bubbles go with everything, especially Asian and fried foods.

The basics of pairing food and wine should be considered when selecting a wine for a meal, but don't let this confine you to one type.

- Don't let the food or wine overwhelm the other—try to maintain a balance between the type of flavors in both the wine and food. Lighter food = lighter wine.
- Think about the ingredients in the dish, not just the main ingredient, such as fish, chicken, etc. Is there acidity, sweetness, or spice? The wine should be paired with the boldest flavor.
- If there is acidity in both the food and wine, the acidity will recede and the other characteristics will come out.

- If there is earth in wine, there should be less in the food or the flavor will be that of dirt. Cheese is one of the most prominent foods that this can happen with.
- Glass shape will help to reveal the wine's best characteristics. For instance, a white wine glass is smaller and more tapered at the top to keep the chill on the wine, while a red wine glass is more open to allow the wine to breathe. A champagne glass is tall and narrow to allow the bubbles to flourish.

Another easy-to-understand pairing tip is this: think about wine in relationship to a standard household item—milk. Wine can be classified by weight; most of us will understand this well. Compare wine to the types of milk we are familiar with, such as skim, 1%, 2%, whole, and cream. Now think of your food in terms of weight and you will be on the road to more interesting pairings.

Also, think about the characteristics of wine and food such as salty, sweet, and acidic. For example, a high-acid salad dressing, your homemade vinaigrette, needs a high-acid wine like Sauvignon Blanc. While vinaigrette can be light, it is still high in acid. Chardonnay would be too "weighty" for vinaigrette and the acid in the dressing would make the Chardonnay taste flat. Think not only about the protein (chicken, beef, fish), but also the sauce that is going on the protein. The sauce ingredients should be considered as well as the protein when selecting your wine.

Some of my favorite pairings are:

- Hors d'oeuvres with Prosecco: an Italian bubbly that is dry, light, and crisp
- Asian food with Prosecco or a light, crisp, dry white, such as Orvieto or Soave from Italy
- Hearty comfort food dishes with red wines
- Roast chicken with rosé
- Mushroom-centric dishes with Pinot Noir
- Osso buco with Barolo or a Piedmontese table wine

A helpful tip for conserving on wine consumption is to alternate sips of wine and water.

My best advice is to TASTE and find out what you like. After a while, you will be able to taste the wine and food in your mind's eye when selecting the appropriate wine. I sometimes will decide on the wine and then select the recipe.

Enjoy!

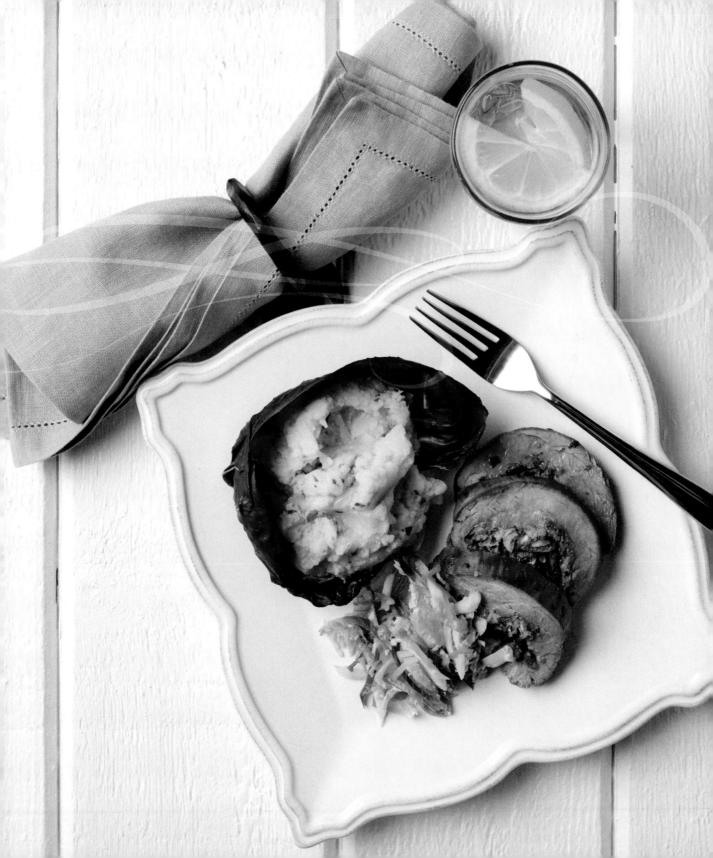

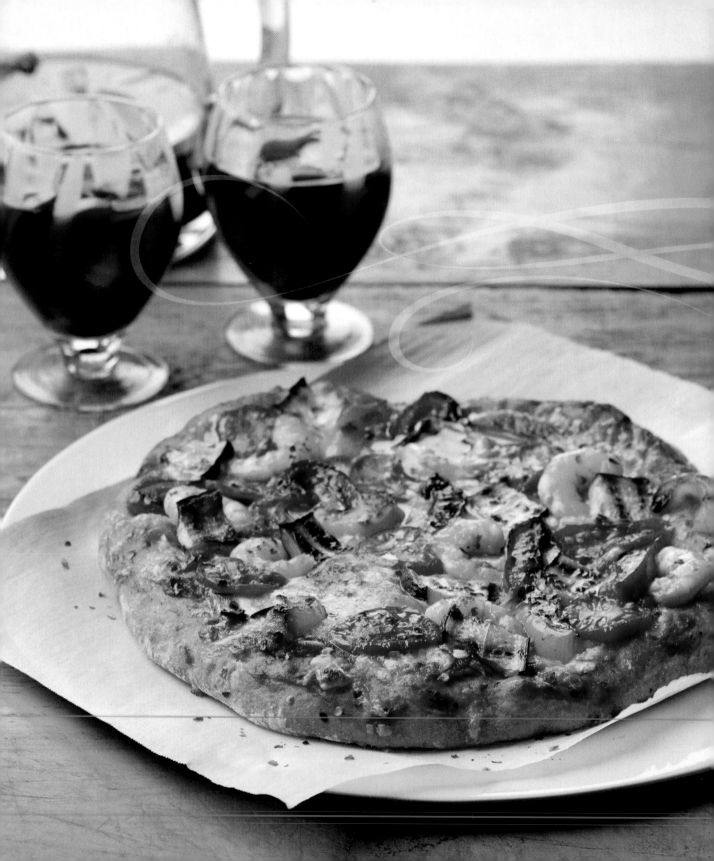

AL FRESCO

Al Fresco

There's nothing quite like grilling outside on a warm summer evening. Al fresco dining usually includes grilling, so here are some Grilling 101 tips so you can have the easiest, most delicious al fresco meals for you and your family.

GRILLING TIPS

Grilling is a wonderful way to cook! It can be quick, easy, healthy, and requires little or no cleanup. It is also a great casual way to entertain. Many folks commonly confuse "grilling" and barbecuing. Barbecue is a slow-cooked piece of meat in a piquant sauce originating in the South. Grilling is much different. Weber-Stephen defines grilling as "an art form that depends largely on controlling the fire, getting the seasonings just right, and mastering a special technique". There are many cultures and cuisines that can be explored through grilling. You can visit many of them through the use of different spices, marinades, and rubs. During the summer months, it is especially nice to cook with what's in season.

There are many different types of grills. It is not necessary to overbuy. Will you use all those bells and whistles? Grilling can be done indoors or outdoors, at your home, at a picnic ground, or at a tailgate location. Are there any restrictions on grills in your community?

The most commonly available grills are:

- Gas grill (outside)—uses lava rocks or flavorizer bars system, sometimes restricted in condo, townhouse, or apartment complexes
- Electric grill (inside or outside)—one sided or two sided, open or closed
- Stovetop grill pan (inside)—round, square, single or double burner, with lid or without
- Charcoal (outside)—uses charcoal briquettes

RECOMMENDED GRILLING TOOLS AND ACCESSORIES

- Spray bottle of water (for safety)
- Long-handled tools, such as tongs, spatulas, etc.
- Meat thermometer
- Basting brush (for marinades)
- Wire brush (for cleaning grill)
- Skewers—metal and wooden
- Rotisserie attachment
- Mitts and potholders
- Disposable foil pans
- Grill cover
- Spare tank of propane gas

SAFETY IS VERY IMPORTANT

- Maintain grill properly (see your owner's manual)
- Keep water nearby
- Do not grill in an area that is not well ventilated
- Do not grill in extremely windy conditions
- Drain marinades and sauces from food before placing on the grill to avoid flareups from the sugars, fats, or oils

HELPFUL HINTS FOR GRILLING

1. Preheat the grill for at least ten minutes or until the inside temperature reaches 500–550°F.
2. Brush the hot grill to clean it (use a metal brush).
3. Keep the cover closed so that the heat circulates evenly and the grill can impart some of the smoky flavor that many expect.
4. Trim visible fat so that there is less fat to drip into the flames causing flareups. Keep a spray bottle of water nearby to spritz any flare-ups.
5. Oil the food, not the grill. The oil will be in the marinade or lightly rubbed on the food.
6. Use tongs to turn your food to avoid piercing the meat and having juices drip into the flames or coals, which causes flareups.
7. Grill presentation side first. Cook food long enough to release itself from the cooking surface to ensure visual appeal.
8. When should food be turned? Turn food only once— wait for caramelization (browning). This means that you don't pry it off the grill. When it is ready, you will be able to turn it easily, leaving nothing behind.
9. When is it done? Use an instant-read meat thermometer and check food frequently to ensure proper sanitation and avoid any bacteria buildup. The minimum internal temperature should be:
    - Poultry—165°
    - Meat (Beef, Lamb, Pork, Veal) Chops & Roasts—Ground 160°F, Roasts, 145°F Med. Rare, 160°F Med., 170°F Well Done
    - Stuffing—165° in center of stuffing
10. Let meat rest before slicing so that the juices do not rush out when the meat is cut or sliced.
11. If you use a gas grill, keep a full spare tank on hand to avoid running out of gas while you are sitting on your deck or patio enjoying your lovely backyard surroundings.
12. The natural sugars in fresh fruits make them a great candidate for grilling. Simply cut up your favorite fruits, place on skewers, and grill until beautifully browned for a light dessert or side dish.
13. Fresh flowers from your garden such as nasturtiums and pansies, which are edible, and fresh herbs, make lovely garnishes for your special summer dishes. Be creative!

RECIPES

Before beginning any cooking process, you should read the recipe thoroughly so that you do not encounter any surprises! There are also some variables to consider, such as wind, outside temperature, the size and shape of your ingredients, and the grill that you are using. Thinking about the particular circumstances can make a huge difference when grilling and also give better results. High-sugar sauces or marinades should be drained from the meat before placing on the grill to avoid flare-ups. They can be lightly brushed on the meat after it has been turned once. Rosemary stems make great skewers because they will impart their flavor into whatever is being "skewered."

I like to use a basic extra virgin olive oil, red wine vinegar, salt, pepper, and fresh herb mixture as a marinade for whatever I am grilling. Reserve some of this to dress your salad and the meal will be simple, fresh, delicious, and harmonious.

Basic Grilled Chicken

1 (6-ounce) boneless, skinless
  chicken breast
1/8 teaspoon fine sea salt
1/8 teaspoon freshly ground pepper

Mastering basic grilled chicken is a very handy tool. From this, you can prepare as many dishes as you can think of. For starters, you can top a green salad, turn it into chicken salad, fill a panini, and so much more. You can be as creative as your imagination will allow.

SERVES 1 | **SERVING SIZE** 1/2 breast | **EXCHANGES** 4 Lean Meat

1. Pound chicken breast to even thickness. This allows for more even cooking. Season both sides with salt and pepper.

2. Preheat grill or grill pan. Grill 3–4 minutes on each side. Do not turn the chicken until it allows you to turn it. If it sticks, it is not ready to be turned.

Cook's Tips

IN ORDER TO AVOID THE CHICKEN STICKING TO THE GRILL OR GRILL PAN, MAKE SURE THE GRILL IS PREHEATED FOR AT LEAST 10 MINUTES.

Calories 190
  Calories from Fat 35
Total Fat 4.0 g
  Saturated Fat 1.2 g
  Trans Fat 0.0 g
Cholesterol 95 mg
Sodium 380 mg
Potassium 295 mg
Total Carbohydrate 0 g
  Dietary Fiber 0 g
  Sugars 0 g
Protein 35 g
Phosphorus 260 mg

Chicken alla Mattone

1 5–6 pound chicken, washed

2 tablespoons of your favorite seasoning blend, such as Italian or Herbs de Provence

1 brick or cast iron pan wrapped in aluminum foil

Chicken Alla Mattone translates to "Chicken under a brick." Cooking your chicken this way produces an extremely crispy skin and very moist meat. It is a fun way to cook chicken and also a conversation starter when your guests see what you are doing. Make this chicken your very own by seasoning it with your favorite flavors. I use an Italian blend of rosemary, basil, garlic, sea salt, and pepper, but you can use whatever you like.

SERVES 8 | SERVING SIZE 1/8 chicken | EXCHANGES 4 Lean Meat

1. Cut chicken through backbone and flatten. Sprinkle skin side with your herb blend.

2. Preheat grill or grill pan. Place on grill skin side down and top with brick or heavy pan. Cook on medium or over indirect heat, depending on your grill, about 45 minutes or until meat thermometer reads 165°F in the thigh.

3. Cut into 8 sections: thighs, legs, wings, and breasts. Remove skin before serving.

Calories 175
  Calories from Fat 65
Total Fat 7.0 g
  Saturated Fat 1.9 g
  Trans Fat 0.0 g
Cholesterol 80 mg
Sodium 80 mg
Potassium 225 mg
Total Carbohydrate 0 g
  Dietary Fiber 0 g
  Sugars 0 g
Protein 26 g
Phosphorus 180 mg

AL FRESCO

Figs Wrapped in Prosciutto

Fresh figs

1 slice of imported prosciutto for each 2 figs

1 teaspoon Gorgonzola cheese for each fig

Calories 60
   Calories from Fat 15
Total Fat 1.5 g
   Saturated Fat 0.8 g
   Trans Fat 0.0 g
Cholesterol 5 mg
Sodium 165 mg
Potassium 150 mg
Total Carbohydrate 10 g
   Dietary Fiber 1 g
   Sugars 8 g
Protein 3 g
Phosphorus 40 mg

SERVES 1 | SERVING SIZE 1 wrapped fig | EXCHANGES 1/2 Fruit, 1/2 Fat

1. Place the prosciutto on the work surface. Place fig in center. Sprinkle 1 teaspoon Gorgonzola around fig. Wrap prosciutto so that cheese is enclosed.

2. Grill on low or bake in the oven until the prosciutto begins to crisp and the cheese softens. Serve as appetizer.

Cook's Tips

THE SIZE OF THE FIGS WILL DETERMINE IF YOU WILL WANT TO USE A WHOLE SLICE OR A HALF SLICE OF PROSCIUTTO PER FIG. YOU WILL WANT ENOUGH PROSCIUTTO TO COMPLETELY WRAP THE FIG. FIGS ARE VERY SOFT TO THE TOUCH WHEN RIPE.

Sautéed Spinach

16 ounces baby spinach

Calories 15
   Calories from Fat 0
Total Fat 0.0 g
   Saturated Fat 0.0 g
   Trans Fat 0.0 g
Cholesterol 0 mg
Sodium 45 mg
Potassium 315 mg
Total Carbohydrate 2 g
   Dietary Fiber 1 g
   Sugars 0 g
Protein 2 g
Phosphorus 30 mg

SERVES 8 | SERVING SIZE 1/8 recipe | EXCHANGES Free Food

1. Rinse the spinach in a colander.

2. Place spinach in a large nonstick skillet. Cook until spinach is tender, about 5 minutes.

Fresh Tomato, Basil, and Cucumber Salad

3 pounds fresh tomatoes

1 teaspoon fine sea salt

2–3 fresh cucumbers (about 2 cups), sliced

2 cloves garlic, finely minced

1 shallot or small onion, minced

2 tablespoons red wine vinegar

1/4 cup extra virgin olive oil

Few turns on the pepper mill

1 cup fresh basil leaves

This salad definitely says summer outdoor dining! Tomatoes and basil are at their best during the summer. Make this salad a few hours ahead so that the flavors will really blend. Consider using a variety of tomatoes for added flavor, color, and nutritional value.

SERVES 7 | SERVING SIZE 1/7 recipe | EXCHANGES 2 Vegetable, 1 1/2 Fat

1. Cut tomatoes into bite-size pieces and place in a large bowl. Sprinkle with salt. Let sit while you prep remaining ingredients.

2. Mix tomatoes, cucumbers, garlic, and shallot. Add vinegar, olive oil, and pepper. Taste for seasoning and adjust seasonings to your liking.

3. Tear basil leaves and add to tomato mixture. Serve at room temperature.

VARIATIONS:
- ADD CHUNKS OF FRESH MOZZARELLA OR YOUR FAVORITE CHEESE
- ADD 1 SMALL SAUTÉED ZUCCHINI

Calories 110
Calories from Fat 70
Total Fat 8.0 g
Saturated Fat 1.1 g
Trans Fat 0.0 g
Cholesterol 0 mg
Sodium 350 mg
Potassium 510 mg
Total Carbohydrate 9 g
Dietary Fiber 3 g
Sugars 5 g
Protein 2 g
Phosphorus 60 mg

Grilled Antipasto with Speck & Asiago

2 small eggplants, cut in half lengthwise

1 small fennel bulb, sliced about 1/4 inch thick

1 small head radicchio, cut into quarters, core intact

1 large Belgian endive, cut in half lengthwise

1 small red onion, sliced into 1/4-inch-thick rounds

1 yellow bell pepper, cut into quarters or rings, seeds removed

1 orange bell pepper, cut into quarters or rings, seeds removed

2 tablespoons extra virgin olive oil

1 medium tomato, sliced

1 ounce sliced speck (about 10 slices)

1 ounce Asiago fresco, cut into bite-size pieces

1 ounce Asiago staggionato, cut into bite-size pieces

6 Cerignola olives (optional)

This is a great plate to share. There is a lot of variety from the vegetable assortment suggested here, but you can also use whatever vegetables are your favorite. Asiago fresco is fresh, unaged Asiago, while Asiago staggionato is aged. This will give a nice contrast in flavor and texture. The aged will be sharp while the fresh will be creamy.

SERVES 4 | **SERVING SIZE** 1/4 recipe | **EXCHANGES** 6 Vegetable, 2 1/2 Fat

1. Lightly salt the cut sides of the eggplants.

2. Place all vegetables except tomato and olives in a large bowl. Add the extra virgin olive oil and toss to coat evenly. Let sit a few minutes while you preheat the grill or grill pan.

3. Grill vegetables to desired doneness and arrange on large platter. Add tomato, speck, Asiago, and finish with olives (if desired).

Cook's Tips

SALTING THE EGGPLANT DRAWS MOISTURE TO THE SURFACE SO THAT IT DOESN'T ABSORB TOO MUCH OIL.

Calories 260
Calories from Fat 115
Total Fat 13.0 g
Saturated Fat 4.3 g
Trans Fat 0.0 g
Cholesterol 20 mg
Sodium 445 mg
Potassium 875 mg
Total Carbohydrate 31 g
Dietary Fiber 9 g
Sugars 12 g
Protein 10 g
Phosphorus 205 mg

AL FRESCO

Grilled Eggplant, Roasted Red Pepper & Mozzarella on Baguette

1 clove fresh garlic, grated on zester

2 tablespoons extra virgin olive oil

1/2 teaspoon fine sea salt (divided use)

1/2 teaspoon freshly ground black pepper

1 medium eggplant, thinly sliced

1 (1-pound) fresh multi-grain Italian baguette

2 Roasted Peppers (see page 20)

4 ounces fresh mozzarella, sliced thinly

Fresh basil leaves

SERVES 8 | **SERVING SIZE** 1/8 recipe
EXCHANGES 1 1/2 Starch, 1 Vegetable, 1 Lean Meat, 1 Fat

1. Mix garlic and 2 tablespoons olive oil together. Add pinch salt and a grinding or two of fresh black pepper.

2. Slice eggplant into 1/4-inch rounds. Sprinkle with remaining salt and let sit a few minutes. When moisture comes to surface, lightly brush with olive oil mixture.

3. Heat grill pan and grill eggplant until fork tender.

4. Slice baguette into two long, thin pieces. Brush with remaining olive oil and grill bread lightly.

5. Layer bottom baguette half with vegetables and mozzarella. Top with basil leaves and remaining baguette half. Press down and cut into 8 individual pieces.

Calories 250
  Calories from Fat 80
Total Fat 9.0 g
  Saturated Fat 2.5 g
  Trans Fat 0.0 g
Cholesterol 5 mg
Sodium 465 mg
Potassium 315 mg
Total Carbohydrate 33 g
  Dietary Fiber 7 g
  Sugars 8 g
Protein 12 g
Phosphorus 205 mg

AL FRESCO

Grilled Eggplant with Spinach Pesto

SPINACH PESTO

4 cups fresh spinach

1 cup fresh parsley

5 tablespoons grated Parmigiano-Reggiano

2 cloves garlic

1/2–1 cup chicken or vegetable stock

2 baby eggplants, white, pink, or purple

1 teaspoon extra virgin olive oil

SERVES 4 | SERVING SIZE 1/2 baby eggplant | EXCHANGES 1 Vegetable, 1/2 Fat

1. Place spinach, parsley, Parmigiano–Reggiano, and garlic in food processor until smooth. Add stock to desired consistency.

2. Cut eggplants in half lengthwise. Brush with olive oil and grill until flesh is soft. You can also bake these in the oven at 400°F for 20–30 minutes.

3. Spread spinach pesto on top of eggplant and garnish with a light sprinkling of Parmigiano.

Calories 70
  Calories from Fat 30
Total Fat 3.5 g
  Saturated Fat 1.5 g
  Trans Fat 0.0 g
Cholesterol 5 mg
Sodium 195 mg
Potassium 340 mg
Total Carbohydrate 7 g
  Dietary Fiber 2 g
  Sugars 2 g
Protein 4 g
Phosphorus 80 mg

AL FRESCO

Grilled Vegetables with Balsamic Drizzle

1 cup balsamic vinegar

GRILLED VEGETABLES

1 large eggplant, unpeeled and sliced into 1/4-inch-thick rounds

1/2 teaspoon fine sea salt

2 medium zucchini, unpeeled and sliced lengthwise 1/4 inch thick

2 sweet onions, peeled and sliced into very thin rounds

1 red bell pepper, cored and sliced into 1/4-inch rounds

1 green bell pepper, cored and sliced into 1/4-inch rounds

1 yellow bell pepper, cored and sliced into 1/4-inch rounds

2 tablespoons extra virgin olive oil

1/2 teaspoon freshly ground pepper

Fresh basil (for garnish)

This vegetable platter makes a lovely centerpiece for a summer buffet table. Consider your grill when slicing vegetables and cut them thick enough so that they will not fall through the grate. Varying the vegetable types and sizes will add to the appearance of your platter. Fresh fruit can also be grilled. The Balsamic Drizzle is a finishing touch but the vegetables are also great by themselves. An edible flower garnish is also a nice touch!

SERVES 8 | SERVING SIZE 1/8 recipe | EXCHANGES 1/2 Carbohydrate, 3 Vegetable, 1/2 Fat

1. Preheat grill.
2. Place vinegar in small saucepan and simmer for 15–20 minutes until reduced to 1/2 cup.
3. Place eggplant in large bowl, add salt, and let sit for 10 minutes. (This will lessen the amount of oil absorbed by the eggplant.)
4. Add remaining vegetables and toss with olive oil and pepper.
5. Place on preheated grill and cook to desired doneness.
6. Drizzle vegetables with balsamic reduction. Garnish with fresh basil sprigs.

Cook's Tips

SOME VEGETABLES ONLY REQUIRE GRILLING ON ONE SIDE.
HEAT KILLS VITAMINS AND MINERALS, SO THE CRISPIER THE BETTER.

THINLY SLICED POTATOES ARE NICE ON THE GRILL.

CAN BE MADE EARLY IN THE DAY AND SERVED AT ROOM TEMPERATURE.

LEFTOVERS CAN BE USED FOR SANDWICHES OR TOSSED WITH PASTA.

Calories 125
   Calories from Fat 35
Total Fat 4.0 g
   Saturated Fat 0.5 g
   Trans Fat 0.0 g
Cholesterol 0 mg
Sodium 165 mg
Potassium 445 mg
Total Carbohydrate 22 g
   Dietary Fiber 4 g
   Sugars 13 g
Protein 2 g
Phosphorus 65 mg

Grilled Pizza

Italian food is an American favorite and pizza most likely leads the list. Making pizza at home is not only fun but creative. You can custom-make your own pizza with the kids or have an adult pizza party. "Put on your bunny slippers, pour a glass of wine, and cook!" Rather than the same old, same old, why not try a grilled pizza? Grilling pizza is really very simple. No pizza pans required, just dependable dough and a hot grill with a lid. Your grill can mimic the pizza ovens found in your favorite pizza shop—on a smaller scale, of course. This dough makes 1 very large (16-inch) pie, 2 medium (8-10 inch) pies, or 4-6 individual pizzas. It can also be used for focaccia.

I recently attended a food conference and enjoyed the lecture given on making pizza at home. The panel consisted of three successful pizzaiolos, all of whom shared their passion for creating a perfect pizza. One thing I took away was that each had their own way of doing things and we can too. Combining their pizza-making skills with their passion, they have created successful pizza businesses while keeping the craft of pizzaiolo alive. A pizzaolo is one dedicated to the craft of pizza perfection. The craft had been dying because chain pizzerias were putting the small shops out of business. Thankfully, we are once again appreciating the artisan pizza maker.

On the suggestion of Brian Spangler of Apizza Scholls in Portland, I have been experimenting with a 24-hour rise, or at least, a longer rise. Dough will double in size in about 90 minutes, which is enough to make a pizza but give it a longer rise and you will have a lighter, bubblier crust. I especially like this for whole-wheat pizza. Whole-wheat flour is heavier than plain white or all-purpose flour since it includes the endosperm or outer germ layer in the milling process. There is a variety of whole-wheat flour that is milled from white wheat rather than red and it yields a lighter whole-wheat flour. As a general rule of thumb, you use one third to one half whole-wheat flour in a recipe; however, with white whole wheat, you can increase the amount used each time, until you achieve the desired consistency in your baked goods. I like using 2 cups white whole-wheat flour and 2 cups all-purpose flour in my pizza dough.

Once you have your dough made and it is rising, you can think about the toppings. Grilled pizza is best when toppings are used sparingly. Too much on top of the pizza can yield a soggy crust. According to Spangler, extreme high heat also yields crispy, airy crust. Since the pizza doesn't have to cook for a long time, you will want high quality, extremely flavorful toppings. My favorite is a Taleggio, tomato, and fresh basil. Taleggio is a soft, creamy washed Italian rind cheese made from cow's milk, a bit "stinky," but so delicious. I use imported organic Prunotto plum tomatoes from Piemonte, Italy. The tomatoes are packed so that they maintain their integrity and taste as fresh as can be. Top with fresh basil and you have pizza perfection. Serve with a fresh green salad with your own freshly made vinaigrette and you have a perfect summer treat.

1 package or 2 1/4 teaspoons dry yeast (rapid rise is not necessary)

2 cups white whole-wheat flour

2 cups all-purpose flour, plus extra for your work surface

1 hearty pinch of fine sea salt

1 1/4–1 1/2 cups tepid water (using a meat or candy thermometer, the water should measure 110–120°F)

1 tablespoon olive oil, plus extra for coating the dough during the rising process

Cornmeal for sprinkling on the pizza peel, if oven baking

TOPPING SUGGESTIONS

2 cups tomatoes or pizza sauce

1/4 pound Taleggio, sliced

1/4 pound mozzarella, shredded or sliced

Grilled vegetables

Sliced mushrooms

Raw peeled shrimp

Asparagus

Proscuitto

EQUIPMENT

Food processor with steel blade

Large work bowl

Pizza wheel

For optional oven baking only—pizza stone and pizza peel or baking sheet without sides

1. Set up food processor with steel blade (an electric mixer fitted with a dough hook also works well). Pour flour, salt, and yeast into food processor. Pulse 2–3 times to mix well.

2. Add tepid water and process until a ball forms inside the work bowl. Add 1 tablespoon extra virgin olive oil. Process 2 minutes. The food processor will do the kneading for you.

3. Dough should not be sticky. If it is, you can add more flour. Add the flour 1/4 cup at a time until dough is no longer sticky and does not stick to your hands. When dough is no longer sticky, place dough in a lightly oiled bowl and turn to coat all sides. Cover with plastic wrap and set in a warm place to rise. Dough should double in size within 1 or 2 hours; the longer it rises, the better.

To Grill Pizza

Preheat grill to high or 500°F. Flatten dough to desired size. Do not add toppings yet. Place flattened pizza dough directly onto grate and cook approximately 3–5 minutes with cover closed, or until grill marks appear and you are able to turn pizza dough with tongs. If it sticks, do not turn it. Give it a few more seconds. Turn dough and add toppings. Close lid and cook another 5 minutes until cheese melts and toppings are cooked.

To Oven Bake Pizza

Preheat oven and pizza stone to 500°F. Prepare pan. To avoid sticking, lightly sprinkle pan with cornmeal or line with parchment paper. If using a pizza peel to transfer pizza to stone, lightly sprinkle the peel with cornmeal. Stretch dough to desired size on pizza peel or prepared pan. Add toppings. Bake in preheated oven until outside edges of crust are golden and cheese is bubbly, approximately 15–20 minutes.

Cook's Tips

TOPPINGS FOR GRILLED PIZZA SHOULD GENERALLY BE LIGHT AND CAN INCLUDE FRESH SLICED TOMATOES, FRESH BASIL FROM YOUR HERB GARDEN, AND FRESH MOZZARELLA. YOU CAN ALSO TOP YOUR PIZZA WITH DOLLOPS OF RICOTTA AND HOMEMADE BASIL MINCED WITH EXTRA VIRGIN OLIVE OIL TO FORM A PASTE.

THE MOISTURE CONTENT IN YOUR FLOUR AND THE ATMOSPHERE IN YOUR KITCHEN CAN VARY GREATLY EACH TIME YOU MAKE PIZZA. THE BEST WAY TO JUDGE THE DOUGH IS BY THE FEEL. IT SHOULD FEEL SMOOTH AND NOT AT ALL STICKY.

LET PIZZA REST 5 MINUTES BEFORE CUTTING, THIS WILL MAKE SLICING EASIER.

A DAMP TEA TOWEL WILL ALSO WORK IN PLACE OF PLASTIC WRAP IF YOU ARE PLACING YOUR DOUGH IN A WARM OVEN (LESS THAN 200 DEGREES) TO RISE. A HOT, HUMID, SUMMER DAY IS GREAT FOR RISING. PLACING THE DOUGH ON TOP OF A WARM STOVE IS ALSO A GOOD METHOD FOR HELPING THE DOUGH RISE.

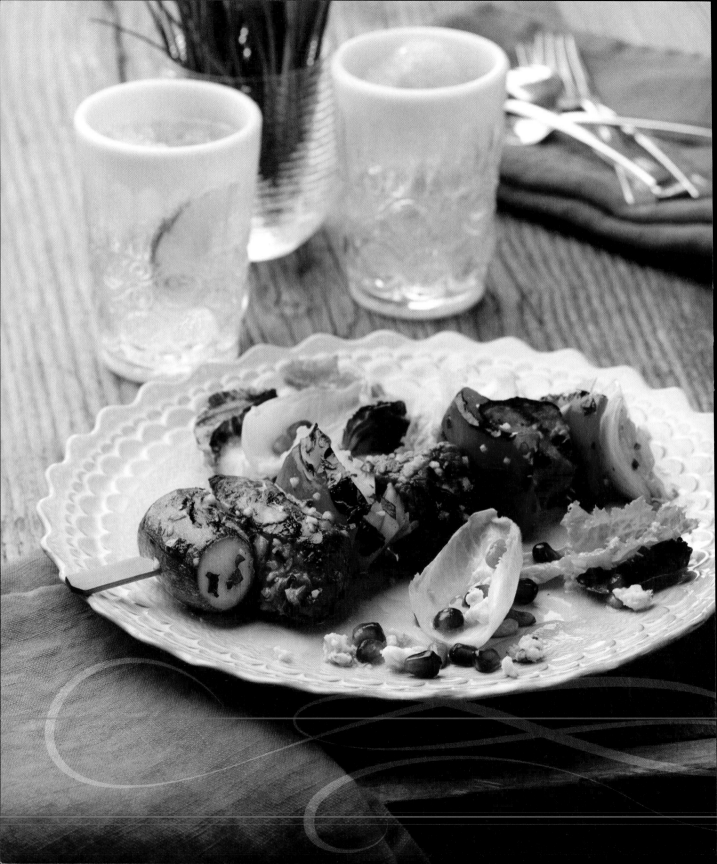

Grilled Lamb Kabobs with Lemon Garlic Vinaigrette

LEMON GARLIC VINAIGRETTE

Juice of 1 lemon

1/4 cup extra virgin olive oil

1 clove garlic, minced

2 tablespoons fresh oregano or 1/2 teaspoon dried oregano

2 pounds boneless leg of lamb, cut into 2-inch pieces

1 medium zucchini, cut into 2-inch pieces

1 small eggplant, cut into 2-inch pieces

1 large red bell pepper, cut into 2-inch pieces

1 medium onion, cut into 2-inch pieces

Wooden skewers soaked at least 30 minutes in water (this will prevent charring)

SERVES 8 | SERVING SIZE 1 skewer | EXCHANGES 2 Vegetable, 3 Lean Meat, 2 Fat

1. Whisk all vinaigrette ingredients together in medium bowl. The vinaigrette will stay together better if whisked rather than shaken.

2. Marinate lamb and vegetables in Lemon Garlic Vinaigrette for at least 1 hour.

3. Preheat grill. Divide vegetables and lamb equally among the 8 skewers. Place on preheated grill.

4. Grill to desired temperature. Serve over Sautéed Spinach (page 6) or a Tre Colore salad (page 24).

Calories 280
  Calories from Fat 135
Total Fat 15.0 g
  Saturated Fat 3.9 g
  Trans Fat 0.0 g
Cholesterol 80 mg
Sodium 75 mg
Potassium 530 mg
Total Carbohydrate 9 g
  Dietary Fiber 2 g
  Sugars 4 g
Protein 26 g
Phosphorus 220 mg

Lime Cilantro Swordfish with Mixed Beans and Pineapple Salsa

SWORDFISH MARINADE

1 tablespoon honey

Juice of 2 limes

1 tablespoon extra virgin olive oil

1/8 teaspoon fine sea salt

Freshly ground black pepper

1 tablespoon chopped fresh cilantro

1 pound swordfish (tuna can also be used)

BEAN AND PINEAPPLE SALSA

1 cup black beans, drained and rinsed

1 cup finely diced fresh pineapple (same size dice as beans)

1/2 teaspoon ground cumin

1 tablespoon extra virgin olive oil

1/2 cup chopped fresh cilantro

Juice of 2 limes

2 tablespoons minced red onion

1/8 teaspoon fine sea salt

Few grinds freshly milled black pepper

SERVES 4 | SERVING SIZE 1/4 recipe
EXCHANGES *(for Lime Cilantro Swordfish only)* 1/2 Carbohydrate, 3 Lean Meat, 1/2 Fat
EXCHANGES *(for Bean and Pineapple Salsa only)* 1/2 Starch, 1/2 Fruit, 1 Fat

1. Mix honey, lime juice, olive oil, pinch sea salt, a few grinds of black pepper, and cilantro together for marinade. Place swordfish in marinade for at least 20 minutes and up to 2 hours.

2. Mix together Bean and Pineapple Salsa ingredients. Prepare the salsa early in the day, if possible, to allow flavors to blend.

3. To cook swordfish: heat grill or sauté pan. Place fish on grill and cook about 3 minutes on first side. Turn and cook to desired doneness on second side.

4. Place a portion of fish on plate and top with salsa. Garnish with fresh cilantro sprigs. (You can also use Mango Kiwi Relish and Strawberry Kiwi Relish as variations.)

Cook's Tips

THE BLACK BEAN SALSA AND MANGO KIWI AND STRAWBERRY KIWI RELISHES ARE ALSO NICE WITH ANY GRILLED PROTEIN.

FOR SWORDFISH	FOR SALSA
Calories 185	*Calories* 115
Calories from Fat 70	*Calories from Fat* 35
Total Fat 8.0 g	*Total Fat* 4.0 g
Saturated Fat 1.7 g	*Saturated Fat* 0.5 g
Trans Fat 0.0 g	*Trans Fat* 0.0 g
Cholesterol 45 mg	*Cholesterol* 0 mg
Sodium 180 mg	*Sodium* 135 mg
Potassium 340 mg	*Potassium* 235 mg
Total Carbohydrate 6 g	*Total Carbohydrate* 17 g
Dietary Fiber 0 g	*Dietary Fiber* 5 g
Sugars 5 g	*Sugars* 5 g
Protein 22 g	*Protein* 4 g
Phosphorus 300 mg	*Phosphorus* 70 mg

Mango Kiwi Relish

1 mango, diced

2 kiwis, chopped

1/4 cup cilantro, roughly chopped

1 orange, juiced

Calories 80
   Calories from Fat 0
Total Fat 0.0 g
   Saturated Fat 0.1 g
   Trans Fat 0.0 g
Cholesterol 0 mg
Sodium 0 mg
Potassium 290 mg
Total Carbohydrate 20 g
   Dietary Fiber 3 g
   Sugars 16 g
Protein 1 g
Phosphorus 25 mg

SERVES 4 | SERVING SIZE 1/4 recipe
EXCHANGES *(for Mango Kiwi Relish only)* 1 1/2 Fruit

1. Mix all ingredients together. If you can make the relish while you are marinating the fish, it will give these flavors a chance to blend as well.

2. Serve with Lime Cilantro Swordfish (page 16) or your favorite fish.

Strawberry Kiwi Relish

1 cup strawberries, diced

2 kiwis, chopped

1/4 cup cilantro, roughly chopped

1 orange, juiced

Calories 55
   Calories from Fat 0
Total Fat 0.0 g
   Saturated Fat 0.0 g
   Trans Fat 0.0 g
Cholesterol 0 mg
Sodium 0 mg
Potassium 255 mg
Total Carbohydrate 13 g
   Dietary Fiber 3 g
   Sugars 9 g
Protein 1 g
Phosphorus 30 mg

SERVES 4 | SERVING SIZE 1/4 recipe
EXCHANGES *(for Strawberry Kiwi Relish only)* 1 Fruit

1. Mix all ingredients together. If you can make the relish while you are marinating the fish, it will give these flavors a chance to blend as well.

2. Serve with Lime Cilantro Swordfish (page 16) or your favorite fish.

Fresh Herb, Lemon & Garlic Cornish Hens

2 Cornish hens or a small chicken (total weight 3 1/2 pounds)

1/2 cup fresh basil leaves

1/2 cup fresh Italian parsley

5–6 fresh garlic cloves, sliced into rounds

1 teaspoon fine sea salt

1 teaspoon freshly ground mixed peppercorns

This dish is simple and elegant as well as versatile. It can be cooked on your grill or in your oven. If Cornish hens are hard to find, you can substitute a small chicken.

SERVES 4 | SERVING SIZE 1/2 Cornish hen | EXCHANGES 5 Lean Meat

1. Clean hens. Cut alongside backbone separating the hen into one big flat bird. (Splitting along the backbone will help keep the breast moist.)

2. Remove basil and parsley from their stems. Mix with garlic slices. Chop the basil and parsley if the leaves are large; otherwise leave them whole.

3. Gently lift skin and tuck basil, parsley, and garlic under skin. Season outside with salt and pepper.

4. You can cook this dish in one of two ways—either on your grill or in your oven.

To Grill Hens

Place skin side up on preheated grill and grill over indirect heat until golden brown and you reach an internal temperature of 165°F, which takes approximately 30 minutes. (Remove skin before eating.)

To Oven Roast Hens

Preheat oven to 400°F. Place hens on parchment–lined baking sheet and roast approximately 45 minutes or until internal temperature reaches 165°F. (Remove skin before eating.)

~**VARIATIONS:**
- ROASTING CHICKEN: SPLIT THROUGH BACKBONE AND FLATTENED.
- INDIVIDUAL CHICKEN PIECES: WILL TAKE ONLY APPROXIMATELY 30 MINUTES TO COOK
- FRESH OR PRESERVED LEMONS CAN BE USED IN ADDITION TO THE HERBS.

Calories 235
   Calories from Fat 65
Total Fat 7.0 g
   Saturated Fat 1.7 g
   Trans Fat 0.0 g
Cholesterol 185 mg
Sodium 145 mg
Potassium 445 mg
Total Carbohydrate 0 g
   Dietary Fiber 0 g
   Sugars 0 g
Protein 41 g
Phosphorus 260 mg

AL FRESCO

Portobello, Eggplant & Tomato Stacks with Parmigiano-Reggiano

1 large eggplant, sliced into 1/4-inch thick rounds

1/3 teaspoon fine sea salt, divided use

Extra virgin olive oil in spray bottle or olive oil nonstick pan spray

4 portobello mushrooms without stems

1–2 large ripe tomatoes (such as beefsteak)

2 ounces fresh mozzarella

1/2 ounce Parmigiano-Reggiano, freshly grated (keep larger piece in refrigerator and freshly grate the cold cheese)

Fresh rosemary sprigs (optional)

Freshly ground black pepper

Fresh basil for garnish

SERVES 4 | **SERVING SIZE** 1 stack | **EXCHANGES** 3 Vegetable, 1 Fat

1. Preheat grill or grill pan.
2. After eggplant is sliced, lightly salt and let sit to bring water to surface. (This will help to reduce the amount of oil absorbed by the eggplant.)
3. Spray both sides of eggplant lightly with olive oil.
4. Scrape gill from mushrooms with spoon. Spray both sides with olive oil.
5. Slice tomatoes and lightly salt.
6. Slice mozzarella into 4 slices and set aside.
7. Grill eggplant and portobellos, about 3–5 minutes.
8. Layer portobello, eggplant, mozzarella, tomato, and top with Parmigiano shavings. Insert rosemary spring through stack for garnish (optional). Garnish with fresh basil sprigs and freshly ground pepper.

Cook's Tips

TO MAKE PARMIGIANO SHAVINGS: USE A GOOD VEGETABLE PEELER AND VERY COLD CHEESE.

Calories 115
Calories from Fat 45
Total Fat 5.0 g
Saturated Fat 2.5 g
Trans Fat 0.0 g
Cholesterol 10 mg
Sodium 550 mg
Potassium 610 mg
Total Carbohydrate 13 g
Dietary Fiber 4 g
Sugars 6 g
Protein 7 g
Phosphorus 180 mg

Roasted Peppers

1 medium red, yellow, orange, or green sweet bell pepper

Roasting bell peppers is very simple and makes all the difference when used in place of jarred. In the summer when your farmer's market has peppers in abundance, you can purchase the box and sit on your deck or patio with a glass of wine and prepare to fill your freezer with freshly roasted peppers. My mom and I used to enjoy an afternoon together with our box of multi-colored peppers and some great conversation.

SERVES 1 | **SERVING SIZE** 1 pepper | **EXCHANGES** 2 Vegetable

1. Place pepper on grill or side of gas burner and cook until charred. Place in plastic bag or covered bowl and let cool until skin blisters, about 15–20 minutes. Peel charred skin off peppers.

2. Cut peppers into desired-size pieces and discard seeds.

3. Use in sandwiches, salads, or antipasto platters.

Cook's Tips

ROAST SEVERAL COLORS OF BELL PEPPERS AND THEN PLACE ON A PLATTER WITH A LIGHT DRIZZLE OF BALSAMIC VINEGAR, A SPRINKLING OF SEA SALT, AND SOME FRESH HERBS, SUCH AS BASIL, PARSLEY, OR OREGANO FOR A SIMPLE SALAD.

Calories 40
Calories from Fat 0
Total Fat 0.0 g
Saturated Fat 0.1 g
Trans Fat 0.0 g
Cholesterol 0 mg
Sodium 0 mg
Potassium 295 mg
Total Carbohydrate 8 g
Dietary Fiber 2 g
Sugars 4 g
Protein 1 g
Phosphorus 35 mg

AL FRESCO

Wild Rice & Chicken Salad

1/2 cup champagne vinegar

1/4 cup chopped fresh thyme, plus additional for garnish

1/2 cup extra virgin olive oil (have extra available, if desired)

1/2 teaspoon fine sea salt

Freshly ground pepper, to taste

1 pound boneless skinless chicken or turkey breast, grilled and diced

2 cups cooked wild rice

1 cup seedless red and green grapes

8 cups baby greens or spinach

This is a great summer main dish salad. It is cooling and a great do-ahead dish for al fresco dining.

SERVES 8 | SERVING SIZE 1/8 recipe
EXCHANGES 1/2 Starch, 1/2 Carbohydrate, 2 Lean Meat, 2 Fat

1. Mix champagne vinegar and thyme. Slowly whisk in olive oil. Season with salt and pepper.

2. Combine chicken, rice, and grapes. Season to taste with salt and pepper. Add dressing to taste. Serve over baby greens with additional thyme as garnish.

Calories 260
  Calories from Fat 135
Total Fat 15.0 g
  Saturated Fat 2.3 g
  Trans Fat 0.0 g
Cholesterol 30 mg
Sodium 225 mg
Potassium 500 mg
Total Carbohydrate 17 g
  Dietary Fiber 2 g
  Sugars 3 g
Protein 15 g
Phosphorus 155 mg

Flank Steak with Herb Stuffing

2 pounds flank steak

STUFFING

2 cups fresh breadcrumbs

2 shallots, finely minced, or 2 cloves garlic, finely minced

1/4 cup fresh Italian parsley

1/2 cup fresh basil

1 cup fresh spinach, chopped

1 cup fresh mushrooms, thinly sliced

1/4 cup fresh oregano

1/2 cup Parmigiano-Reggiano (optional)

1/4–1/2 cup dry Italian red wine, such as Chianti or Sangiovese

MARINADE

1 cup dry red wine, such as Chianti or Sangiovese

1/4 cup olive oil

2 garlic cloves, crushed

1 teaspoon fine sea salt

1 teaspoon freshly ground pepper

1 tablespoon Worcestershire sauce

GARNISH

Additional fresh herbs

Nasturtium flowers (edible flowers)

Many years ago, I won a cooking contest with this recipe–which I owe to a dear friend for giving me the idea. Garnish with edible flowers such as nasturtiums for a very special presentation. Better grocery stores will have edible flowers in the produce department or you can grow your own!

SERVES 8 | SERVING SIZE 1/8 recipe
EXCHANGES 1/2 Carbohydrate, 3 Lean Meat, 1 Fat

1. Cut the flank steak into 2 thin steaks with a long, thin knife.

2. Mix all stuffing ingredients together and spread over each piece of flank steak. Roll and tie.

3. Mix all marinade ingredients together. Place flank steaks in plastic bag and add marinade. Marinate in the refrigerator for several hours.

4. Preheat grill or grill pan. Drain marinade from steaks.

5. Grill to desired doneness. Slice into very thin rounds and place on platter and garnish with fresh herbs and nasturtium flowers. Can also be served with Mushroom Sherry Sauce (see page 167.)

Cook's Tips

IF TIME PERMITS, MARINATE THE UNSTUFFED MEAT OVERNIGHT INSTEAD.

Calories 225
  Calories from Fat 90
Total Fat 10.0 g
  Saturated Fat 2.9 g
  Trans Fat 0.0 g
Cholesterol 60 mg
Sodium 270 mg
Potassium 410 mg
Total Carbohydrate 8 g
  Dietary Fiber 1 g
  Sugars 1 g
Protein 24 g
Phosphorus 205 mg

AL FRESCO

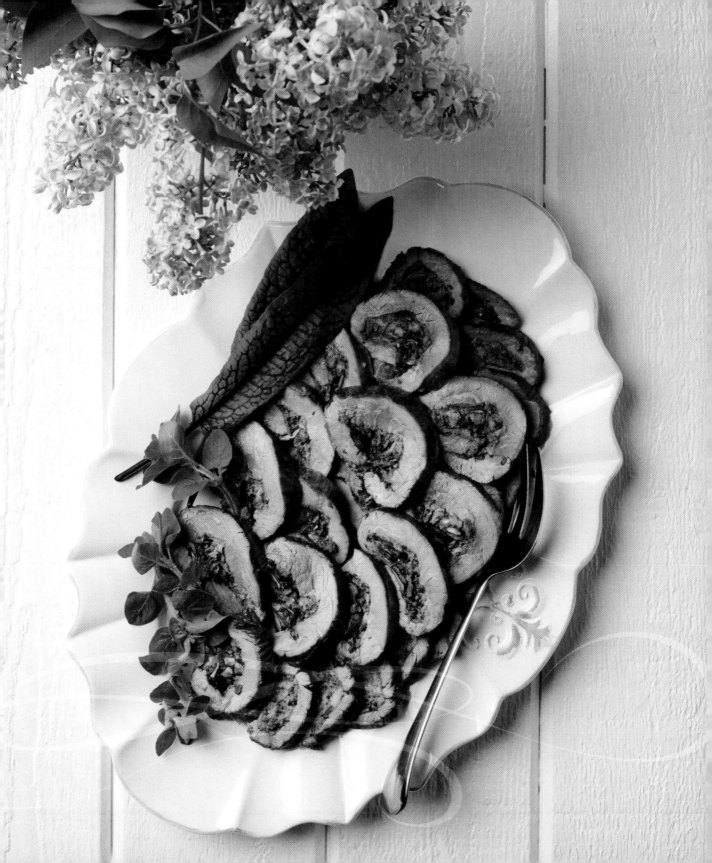

Tre Colore Salad with Vinaigrette

1 head green leaf lettuce

1 small head radicchio

1 medium head Belgian endive or 1 small bunch arugula

1 recipe Basic Vinaigrette (page 173)

EQUIPMENT

Large salad bowl

Salad spinner (optional)

SERVES 4 | SERVING SIZE 1/4 recipe | EXCHANGES 1 Vegetable, 1 Fat

1. Wash and dry salad ingredients. Tear and place in large salad bowl.

2. Add Vinaigrette (page 173) in small amounts and toss well.

VARIATIONS:
- USE A VARIETY OF GREENS, SPRING MIX, OR BABY SPINACH.
- ADD CHEESES AND NUTS THAT COMPLEMENT THE REST OF THE MEAL.

Cook's Tips

SALAD SHOULD NOT BE SWIMMING IN DRESSING. IT'S BETTER TO ADD LESS AND DECIDE YOU NEED MORE.

DRYING THE GREENS IN A SALAD SPINNER HELPS THE DRESSING CLING TO THE GREENS.

Calories 60
Calories from Fat 40
Total Fat 4.5 g
Saturated Fat 0.7 g
Trans Fat 0.0 g
Cholesterol 0 mg
Sodium 35 mg
Potassium 280 mg
Total Carbohydrate 4 g
Dietary Fiber 2 g
Sugars 1 g
Protein 2 g
Phosphorus 35 mg

AL FRESCO

Mock Sangria

4 cups no-sugar-added cranberry pomegranate juice

2 cups seltzer or sparkling mineral water

1 orange, juiced

1 lemon, juiced

1 orange, quartered and sliced

1 lemon, quartered and sliced

1 apple, diced

SERVES 13 | **SERVING SIZE** 1/2 cup | **EXCHANGES** 1 Fruit

1. Mix all ingredients together early in the day and serve with ice in a wine glass.

Calories 45
  Calories from Fat 0
Total Fat 0.0 g
  Saturated Fat 0.1 g
  Trans Fat 0.0 g
Cholesterol 0 mg
Sodium 10 mg
Potassium 60 mg
Total Carbohydrate 11 g
  Dietary Fiber 0 g
  Sugars 11 g
Protein 0 g
Phosphorus 10 mg

AL FRESCO

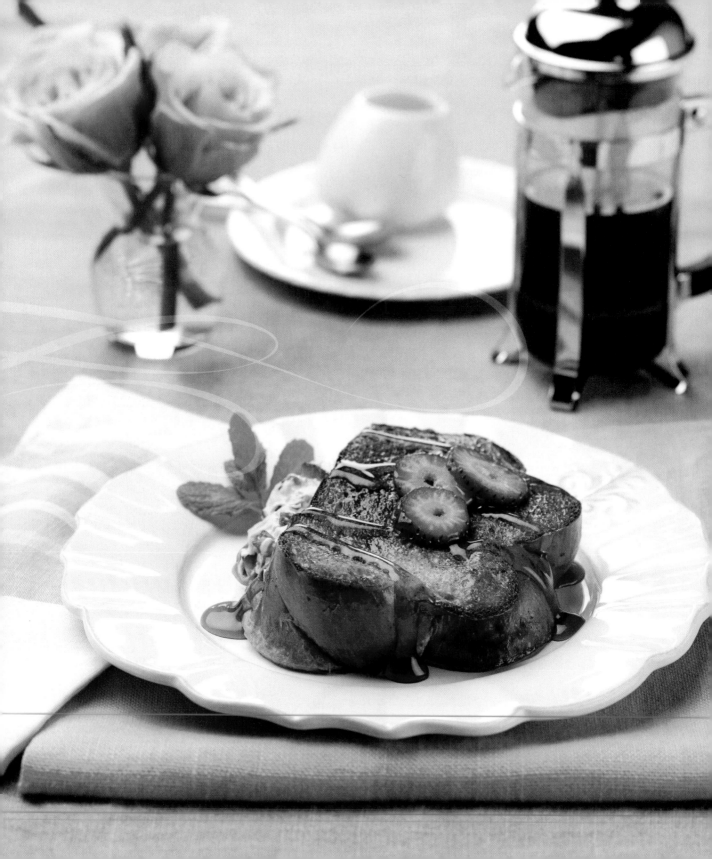

BRUNCH

Apple Compote

2 tablespoons unsalted butter

4 Granny Smith apples, peeled, quartered, and sliced thinly

1 teaspoon ground cinnamon

2 tablespoons honey

1/4 cup water

This warm apple compote will be delicious on so many dishes. Try it on pancakes, waffles, ricotta cheese, frozen yogurt, or in a phyllo dessert shell. If you have a hand-cranked apple peeler, it is perfect for this dish.

SERVES 12 | **SERVING SIZE** 1/3 cup | **EXCHANGES** 1/2 Carbohydrate

1. Melt butter in large sauté pan. Add apples, cinnamon, honey, and water and cook 5–7 minutes until apples are tender.

2. Serve warm or prepare a day or two ahead and reheat at serving time.

Calories 45
  Calories from Fat 20
Total Fat 2.0 g
  Saturated Fat 1.2 g
  Trans Fat 0.0 g
Cholesterol 5 mg
Sodium 0 mg
Potassium 40 mg
Total Carbohydrate 8 g
  Dietary Fiber 1 g
  Sugars 7 g
Protein 0 g
Phosphorus 5 mg

Asparagus with Hollandaise Sauce

2 pounds asparagus, washed and trimmed

HOLLANDAISE SAUCE

2 tablespoons lemon juice

1 tablespoon melted butter

1 cup plain yogurt

1/2 teaspoon fine sea salt

2 eggs or 4 egg whites

I love this dish on a brunch table, but it is a great way to make any meal special.

SERVES 8 | SERVING SIZE 3 tablespoons | **EXCHANGES** 1/2 Carbohydrate, 1/2 Fat

1. Steam asparagus to desired tenderness.
2. Whisk all sauce ingredients in a saucepan. Heat to medium and whisk until mixture barely begins to boil. Remove from heat.
3. Serve warm or chilled over asparagus.

Cook's Tips

FOR A LIGHT MEAL, ADD A POACHED EGG.

Calories 60
  Calories from Fat 25
Total Fat 3.0 g
  Saturated Fat 1.4 g
  Trans Fat 0.1 g
Cholesterol 50 mg
Sodium 205 mg
Potassium 215 mg
Total Carbohydrate 5 g
  Dietary Fiber 1 g
  Sugars 3 g
Protein 4 g
Phosphorus 105 mg

Black Bean and Sweet Potato Hash

4 cups (4 medium) diced sweet potatoes, unpeeled

6 slices turkey bacon, cut into 1-inch pieces

1/2 cup chopped onion

1 large bell pepper, red, yellow, or green, cut into 1/2-inch dice

3/4 teaspoon fine sea salt

15 ounces canned black beans, drained and rinsed well

Freshly ground pepper

This recipe can be served as a brunch item, a side dish to simple grilled meat, or a vegetarian entrée. Carefully read all packages of turkey bacon to find the lowest-fat version. There is a broad range of fat content.

SERVES 6 | SERVING SIZE 1/6 recipe | EXCHANGES 2 Starch, 1/2 Fat

1. Microwave potatoes until almost tender.

2. In sauté pan, cook bacon, onion, bell pepper, potatoes, and a pinch of sea salt over medium-high heat until vegetables are tender and browned. Add beans and cook 5 minutes. Season with pepper.

3. Keep warm until ready to serve.

Cook's Tips

TOP WITH A POACHED EGG FOR ADDED PROTEIN. LOOK FOR "HEALTHIER" EGGS IN THE MARKET THAT HAVE LOWER CHOLESTEROL CONTENT BECAUSE THE HENS ARE FED A BETTER DIET.

Calories 185
Calories from Fat 20
Total Fat 2.5 g
Saturated Fat 0.8 g
Trans Fat 0.0 g
Cholesterol 10 mg
Sodium 565 mg
Potassium 720 mg
Total Carbohydrate 33 g
Dietary Fiber 8 g
Sugars 9 g
Protein 8 g
Phosphorus 155 mg

Fruit & Honey Breakfast Spread

1/2 cup low-fat ricotta cheese

1/2 cup chopped fresh fruit—
  berries, bananas, and apples

1/4 cup raisins or chopped dried
  fruit

2 teaspoons honey

Serve on your favorite bagels, muffins, waffles, or pancakes.

SERVES 5 | **SERVING SIZE** 1/4 cup | **EXCHANGES** 1 Carbohydrate

1. Mix all ingredients in a small bowl.

VARIATIONS: USE YOUR FAVORITE FRESH OR DRIED FRUIT.

Cook's Tips

BEST MADE SEVERAL HOURS AHEAD SO THAT FLAVORS CAN BLEND.

Calories 60
  Calories from Fat 10
Total Fat 1.0 g
  Saturated Fat 0.6 g
  Trans Fat 0.0 g
Cholesterol 5 mg
Sodium 35 mg
Potassium 95 mg
Total Carbohydrate 11 g
  Dietary Fiber 1 g
  Sugars 9 g
Protein 3 g
Phosphorus 55 mg

Broccoli, Mushroom, and Cheddar Omelet

2 whole eggs

4 egg whites

1/4 teaspoon fine sea salt

1/8 teaspoon freshly ground pepper

1/2 teaspoon extra virgin olive oil

1/4 cup chopped onion

1/2 cup sliced mushrooms

1 cup frozen chopped broccoli,
  thawed

Nonstick cooking spray

1 1/2 tablespoons reduced-fat
  cheddar cheese (I used Sargento)

An omelet makes a great brunch as well as a light entrée for lunch or dinner.

SERVES 2 | SERVING SIZE 1/2 omelet | EXCHANGES 1 Vegetable, 2 Lean Meat, 1 Fat

1. Place eggs and egg whites in a large bowl and whisk until light. Add sea salt and pepper.

2. Place olive oil in a medium nonstick sauté pan. Add onion and mushrooms and sauté until onion is translucent and mushrooms are softened. Add broccoli and heat thoroughly. Remove and set aside.

3. Dry the pan. Spray with nonstick cooking spray.

4. Add egg mixture and cook until almost set.

5. Return vegetables to center of eggs. Top with cheddar cheese. Fold over and continue to cook until eggs are done.

~ **VARIATIONS:** USE YOUR FAVORITE VEGETABLES.

Cook's Tips

TWO EGG WHITES ARE THE EQUIVALENT OF ONE WHOLE EGG.

A NONSTICK PAN REALLY HELPS WHEN MAKING AN OMELET, BUT IF YOU DON'T HAVE ONE, YOU CAN LIGHTLY SPRAY YOUR PAN WITH NONSTICK COOKING SPRAY AND WATCH IT VERY CAREFULLY, COOKING ON LOW TO MEDIUM.

Calories 165
  Calories from Fat 65
Total Fat 7.0 g
  Saturated Fat 2.4 g
  Trans Fat 0.0 g
Cholesterol 190 mg
Sodium 530 mg
Potassium 435 mg
Total Carbohydrate 7 g
  Dietary Fiber 3 g
  Sugars 3 g
Protein 18 g
Phosphorus 200 mg

BRUNCH

Dylan's Blueberry Muffins

1 cup Splenda

4 egg whites

1 teaspoon vanilla extract

12 ounces plain, nonfat yogurt

2 cups all-purpose flour

1 tablespoon baking powder

1 cup blueberries

1 tablespoon flour (to coat blueberries)

Nonstick pan coating

EQUIPMENT

Cupcake pan and cupcake liners

I created this recipe for my nephew who was on a NO FAT diet. He really loved them!

SERVES 12 | **SERVING SIZE** 1 muffin | **EXCHANGES** 1 1/2 Carbohydrate

1. Preheat oven to 350°F.

2. In a large bowl, combine Splenda, egg whites, and vanilla. Mix completely. Add yogurt.

3. Combine flour and baking powder. Slowly add to above, until well blended.

4. Add blueberries that have been lightly coated with flour. Mix well.

5. Coat cupcake pans with nonstick pan coating. Fill cupcake pans to top with batter.

6. Bake for 30 minutes until tops are golden or until toothpick comes out clean.

Calories 115
  Calories from Fat 0
Total Fat 0.0 g
  Saturated Fat 0.1 g
  Trans Fat 0.0 g
Cholesterol 0 mg
Sodium 130 mg
Potassium 115 mg
Total Carbohydrate 22 g
  Dietary Fiber 1 g
  Sugars 5 g
Protein 5 g
Phosphorus 185 mg

BRUNCH

Mushroom Frittata with Pancetta & Tomato

1 teaspoon extra virgin olive oil

1 ounce finely diced pancetta
(Italian bacon)

1/4 cup diced onion, about 1 small

4 ounces cremini mushrooms,
sliced

1 cup grape tomatoes, sliced in half
vertically

4 large eggs

4 egg whites

Asiago cheese (optional)

When I have weekend guests I love serving this dish. It is very easy to make but looks and tastes like so much more work. Use whatever vegetables you have on hand to make it your own.

SERVES 4 | SERVING SIZE 1/4 frittata | EXCHANGES 1 Vegetable, 1 Med-Fat Meat, 1 Fat

1. Place olive oil in large nonstick sauté pan. Add pancetta, onion, and mushrooms. Cook until onion is translucent and mushrooms are wilted. Add tomatoes and mix well. (You do not really cook the tomatoes but warm them.)

2. Scramble eggs and egg whites in large bowl. Pour eggs into pan. As they begin to cook, pick up sides of cooked egg and let the uncooked egg slide underneath. Repeat until there is no liquid egg in the pan.

3. Sprinkle with Asiago cheese, if desired. Cover and let cheese melt. Cut into 4 wedges and serve.

Calories 140
  Calories from Fat 70
Total Fat 8.0 g
  Saturated Fat 2.5 g
  Trans Fat 0.0 g
Cholesterol 190 mg
Sodium 260 mg
Potassium 405 mg
Total Carbohydrate 5 g
  Dietary Fiber 1 g
  Sugars 2 g
Protein 12 g
Phosphorus 185 mg

Grilled Salmon with Asparagus & Lemon Sauce

2 pounds asparagus, washed and trimmed

LEMON SAUCE

2 tablespoons lemon juice

1 cup nonfat, plain yogurt

1/2 teaspoon fine sea salt

EQUIPMENT

4-quart saucepan

Vegetable steamer

6 portions of salmon (about 1 1/2 pounds of salmon fillet)

Salt

Pepper

SERVES 6 | SERVING SIZE 1/6 recipe | EXCHANGES 1/2 Carbohydrate, 4 Lean Meat, 1/2 Fat

1. Steam asparagus to desired tenderness.

2. Whisk lemon juice, yogurt, and salt in a small glass bowl. Let sit while preparing the salmon.

3. Preheat grill pan. Sprinkle salmon lightly with sea salt and pepper. Place on preheated grill pan and cook to desired doneness. Turn after first side has been cooking for 3 minutes.

4. Serve warm or chilled with asparagus and sauce.

Calories 235
  Calories from Fat 90
Total Fat 10.0 g
  Saturated Fat 1.8 g
  Trans Fat 0.0 g
Cholesterol 80 mg
Sodium 295 mg
Potassium 610 mg
Total Carbohydrate 6 g
  Dietary Fiber 2 g
  Sugars 4 g
Protein 29 g
Phosphorus 360 mg

Harvest Muffins

2 1/2 cups whole-wheat flour

1 1/2 cups white flour

1 cup sugar

4 teaspoons baking soda

4 teaspoons cinnamon

1/2 teaspoon cloves

1/2 teaspoon nutmeg

4 cups (about 5) finely chopped
unpeeled apples

1 cup (about 3) finely chopped
unpeeled carrots

1 cup raisins

2 cups nonfat yogurt

1/2 cup skim milk

4 teaspoons vanilla extract

4 whole eggs or 8 whites

EQUIPMENT

Large mixing bowls

Muffin tins

Food processor with shredding disk

This is a healthy muffin recipe and is also great as a brunch cake. They are a lovely addition to any meal and they are also a terrific breakfast to go. Try making the cake in a flower-shaped bundt pan such as the rose or chrysanthemum and simply sprinkle with confectioners sugar to enhance the flower petals.

SERVES 36 | **SERVING SIZE** 1 muffin | **EXCHANGES** 1 1/2 Carbohydrate

1. Preheat oven to 350°F.

2. Combine flour, sugar, baking soda, cinnamon, cloves, and nutmeg in a 4-quart bowl.

3. Shred apples and carrots in a food processor with a shredding disk.

4. Add apples, carrots, and raisins to dry ingredients.

5. Mix yogurt, milk, vanilla, and eggs with flour mixture.

6. Prepare pan by either spraying with a nonstick flour spray or spreading with butter and then sprinkling with flour. Discard any excess flour. Fill pans 3/4 full.

7. Bake as follows:
   Mini–20 minutes (yield 72)
   Regular–25–30 minutes (yield 36)
   Large–35-45 minutes (yield 18)
   Cake–60 minutes

Cook's Tips

THIS RECIPE KEEPS WELL BUT MUST BE REFRIGERATED OR FROZEN AFTER 1 DAY DUE TO THE USE OF THE YOGURT.

THESE MUFFINS ARE VERY MOIST SO YOU DON'T NEED TO LINE THE MUFFIN TINS WITH BAKE CUPS. IF YOU CHOOSE TO LINE THE MUFFIN TINS, ALUMINUM, RATHER THAN PAPER BAKE CUPS ARE SUGGESTED.

FOR BREAKFAST TO GO, FREEZE MUFFINS IN INDIVIDUAL BAGGIES.

Calories 110
Calories from Fat 10
Total Fat 1.0 g
Saturated Fat 0.2 g
Trans Fat 0.0 g
Cholesterol 20 mg
Sodium 165 mg
Potassium 155 mg
Total Carbohydrate 24 g
Dietary Fiber 2 g
Sugars 12 g
Protein 3 g
Phosphorus 80 mg

BRUNCH

Portobello Mushrooms Florentine

2 portobello mushroom caps without stems (about 2 ounces each)

1/2 teaspoon extra virgin olive oil

Pinch of salt

4 cups fresh baby spinach

2 large eggs

1 plum tomato, sliced thinly

1 tablespoon grated Grana Padano cheese

I think of this dish as a wonderful romantic breakfast for a special day, but if you want to make it for a crowd you can grill the portobello a day ahead. The spinach-egg mixture takes no time to prepare!

SERVES 2 | **SERVING SIZE** 1/2 recipe | **EXCHANGES** 2 Vegetable, 1 Med-Fat Meat, 1/2 Fat

1. Using a teaspoon, "wipe" the gills from the underside of the mushroom. Brush mushrooms with the extra virgin olive oil and sprinkle with the salt.

2. Heat a grill pan. Grill the mushrooms on the top side first, until you see grill marks. Turn and grill until they begin to soften.

3. Rinse the spinach (even if the package says that it is washed). The water will help to cook the spinach. Place the drained spinach in a medium sauté pan. Cook until spinach begins to wilt. Divide spinach into 2 piles. Crack an egg over each pile. Cook until it begins to set and then turn the egg and spinach over to continue cooking the egg.

4. Top the grilled portobello with this mixture. Top this with sliced tomatoes and sprinkle with cheese. Serve immediately.

Calories 140
  Calories from Fat 65
Total Fat 7.0 g
  Saturated Fat 2.5 g
  Trans Fat 0.0 g
Cholesterol 190 mg
Sodium 335 mg
Potassium 1040 mg
Total Carbohydrate 8 g
  Dietary Fiber 3 g
  Sugars 2 g
Protein 12 g
Phosphorus 255 mg

Quickie Quiche

Nonstick cooking spray

1 1/4 cups 2% evaporated milk

1/4 cup nonfat, plain yogurt

1 teaspoon Dijon mustard

2 large eggs

4 large egg whites

1/2 cup shredded, reduced-fat
Swiss cheese (I use Sargento)

1/4 cup chopped chives

1/2 pound fresh asparagus,
steamed until fork tender

Few grinds fresh black pepper

Additional herbs (for garnish)

EQUIPMENT

8-inch pie plate or 6 individual
ramekins or cupcake pan

Balloon whisk

Large mixing bowl

Small bowls for separating eggs

This recipe is a basic low-fat quiche recipe that you can change as you like. Here we are using low-fat Swiss and asparagus as our guideline, but you can change it each time you make it. I think another great combination would be broccoli and low-fat mozzarella.

SERVES 8 | SERVING SIZE 1/8 recipe | EXCHANGES 1/2 Reduced-Fat Milk, 1 Lean Meat

1. Preheat oven to 350°F. Place rack in center of oven. Spray baking dish with nonstick cooking spray.

2. Mix together milk, yogurt, mustard, eggs, and egg whites until well blended. Add cheese, chives, and asparagus. Blend well.

3. Pour into baking dish(es). Sprinkle with black pepper and additional herbs.

4. Bake until knife inserted in center comes out clean, approximately 35 minutes for one quiche and 20–25 for individuals. Let rest 10–15 minutes before serving. Leftovers can be eaten warm or cold.

Calories 90
Calories from Fat 30
Total Fat 3.5 g
Saturated Fat 1.5 g
Trans Fat 0.0 g
Cholesterol 55 mg
Sodium 120 mg
Potassium 235 mg
Total Carbohydrate 6 g
Dietary Fiber 0 g
Sugars 5 g
Protein 9 g
Phosphorus 165 mg

BRUNCH

Salmon & Chive Pinwheels

8 ounces smoked salmon, thinly sliced

4 ounces light cream cheese (aka Neufchatel, 1/3 less fat)

2 tablespoons chives, snipped or chopped

Additional chopped chives, for garnish

SERVES 12 | **SERVING SIZE** 2 pieces | **EXCHANGES** 1 Lean Meat

1. Lay salmon out so that you have 2 squares, approximately 4 ounces each. It is like making a puzzle.

2. Mix cream cheese and chives together and spread 1/2 of this mixture on each square of salmon.

3. Roll like a jellyroll and freeze for 30 minutes. This will make slicing easier.

4. Mark 24 slices before beginning. Slice with a serrated knife and place on serving platter. Garnish with chopped fresh chives.

5. Serve immediately or cover tightly and refrigerate.

Calories 45
  Calories from Fat 25
Total Fat 3.0 g
  Saturated Fat 1.4 g
  Trans Fat 0.0 g
Cholesterol 10 mg
Sodium 190 mg
Potassium 50 mg
Total Carbohydrate 0 g
  Dietary Fiber 0 g
  Sugars 0 g
Protein 4 g
Phosphorus 45 mg

BRUNCH

Savory Breakfast Casserole

Nonstick cooking spray

4 eggs and 8 egg whites

1/4 teaspoon freshly ground pepper

2 cups skim milk

1 teaspoon Dijon mustard

1 pound vegetarian breakfast sausage, cooked and crumbled

2 slices good-quality whole-grain bread, torn into small pieces

1/2 cup low-fat shredded cheddar cheese (I use Cabot 50% less fat)

This dish is excellent for large groups and can be made ahead because it freezes beautifully.

SERVES 8 | **SERVING SIZE** 1/8 recipe | **EXCHANGES** 1 Carbohydrate, 3 Lean Meat, 1/2 Fat

1. Spray a 9 × 13– inch casserole dish with nonstick spray.
2. Place eggs and pepper in a large mixing bowl. Beat well with a wire whisk. Add milk and mustard. Beat well.
3. Place crumbled sausage and torn bread in bottom of casserole dish. Pour egg–milk mixture over. Sprinkle with cheese.
4. Cover and refrigerate at least 30 minutes or overnight.
5. Preheat oven to 350°F. Bake 30–40 minutes or until set. Casserole will be puffed in the center. Cut into squares and serve hot.

Cook's Tips

REHEATS WELL IN MICROWAVE.

Calories 230
Calories from Fat 70
Total Fat 8.0 g
Saturated Fat 2.4 g
Trans Fat 0.0 g
Cholesterol 100 mg
Sodium 595 mg
Potassium 390 mg
Total Carbohydrate 11 g
Dietary Fiber 2 g
Sugars 5 g
Protein 27 g
Phosphorus 325 mg

Slow-Cooked Oatmeal with Cranberries & Walnuts

1 cup oats (not quick cooking)

1 cup dried fruit, such as cranberries, figs, or apricots

1 cup chopped walnuts

4 cups water

Oatmeal with trimmings is a welcome addition to a brunch buffet. Here's a way to include it without having to prepare it at the last minute. Anything you can include on the menu that can be made ahead of time when entertaining is a must!

SERVES 4 | **SERVING SIZE** 1/4 recipe | **EXCHANGES** 1 Starch, 1 1/2 Fruit, 2 Fat

1. Place all ingredients in your slow cooker. Cover and cook on low for 8 hours. Mix well before serving.

Cook's Tips

THIS CAN BE TURNED ON JUST BEFORE GOING TO BED THE NIGHT BEFORE.

Calories 275
  Calories from Fat 110
Total Fat 12.0 g
  Saturated Fat 1.3 g
  Trans Fat 0.0 g
Cholesterol 0 mg
Sodium 10 mg
Potassium 380 mg
Total Carbohydrate 40 g
  Dietary Fiber 6 g
  Sugars 20 g
Protein 6 g
Phosphorus 160 mg

Strawberry Banana Stuffed French Toast

1 loaf unsliced dense bread (such as challah)

1 pint strawberries, chopped

1 banana, chopped

2 ounces whipped cream cheese

1 cup fat-free ricotta cheese

Nonstick cooking spray

1 1/2 cups egg substitute

1 1/2 cups skim milk

2 teaspoons vanilla extract

3/4 teaspoons ground nutmeg

This is an elegant, easy, make–ahead brunch dish. It can be assembled the day before baking and refrigerated so that you have less work in the morning. I developed this recipe after enjoying a similar dish at a bed & breakfast.

SERVES 6 | SERVING SIZE 1 slice French Toast
EXCHANGES 2 1/2 Starch, 1/2 Fruit, 1/2 Fat-Free Milk, 1 Lean Meat, 1 Fat

1. Cut off a very thin slice at each end of the loaf of bread, then cut into six slices (each about 1 1/2–inch thick). Cut a pocket in each slice.

2. Mix fruit, cream cheese, and ricotta cheese. Stuff each pocket with this mixture.

3. Spray a 9 × 13–inch pan with nonstick cooking spray. Place stuffed bread in pan.

4. Mix egg substitute, milk, vanilla, and nutmeg. Pour over bread.

5. Refrigerate several hours or overnight.

6. Bake at 350°F for approximately 30 minutes until golden.

Calories 355
Calories from Fat 65
Total Fat 7.0 g
Saturated Fat 2.6 g
Trans Fat 0.0 g
Cholesterol 60 mg
Sodium 575 mg
Potassium 485 mg
Total Carbohydrate 52 g
Dietary Fiber 3 g
Sugars 12 g
Protein 21 g
Phosphorus 250 mg

BRUNCH

Strawberry Orange Salad with Lemon Honey Mint Dressing

SALAD

1 pint strawberries

1 large navel orange

1 banana, sliced and dipped in lemon juice

Juice of 1 lemon

Small head green leaf lettuce

DRESSING

1/2 cup nonfat, plain yogurt

1 1/2 teaspoons fresh squeezed orange juice

1 1/2 teaspoons lemon juice (Meyer lemons, if available)

1 tablespoon honey

2 tablespoons minced fresh mint (for garnish)

This salad screams "brunch on the patio" to me.

SERVES 4 | SERVING SIZE 1/4 recipe | **EXCHANGES** 1 1/2 Fruit, 1/2 Carbohydrate

1. Slice strawberries, section orange, and slice banana and dip in lemon juice. Mix together in bowl.

2. Wash and spin-dry the lettuce, keeping leaves as large as possible. Place lettuce equally on each of 4 plates. Divide fruit among 4 lettuce-lined plates. For family style presentation, place lettuce on platter and top with fruit.

3. Mix all dressing ingredients together and spoon over salad plates.

Calories 115
  Calories from Fat 5
Total Fat 0.5 g
  Saturated Fat 0.1 g
  Trans Fat 0.0 g
Cholesterol 0 mg
Sodium 35 mg
Potassium 490 mg
Total Carbohydrate 28 g
  Dietary Fiber 4 g
  Sugars 19 g
Protein 3 g
Phosphorus 95 mg

Waffles

1 large egg

1 3/4 cups 1% milk

1/4 cup canola oil

1 3/4 cups all-purpose flour

1 tablespoon baking powder

1/2 teaspoon salt

2 large egg whites

Special occasions call for special dishes like waffles that might have one extra step than we have time for on the average morning.

SERVES 6 | **SERVING SIZE** 1 waffle | **EXCHANGES** 2 Starch, 2 Fat

1. Mix together whole egg, milk, and canola oil in a small bowl.

2. Whisk together the flour, baking powder, and salt in a large bowl.

3. Beat egg whites with an electric mixer until stiff peaks form.

4. Add egg mixture from small bowl to large bowl. Carefully mix in egg whites by hand. Do not overmix or you will flatten the egg whites.

5. Preheat waffle iron. Depending on size of waffle iron, pour enough batter in to coat the surface. Close waffle iron and cook until steam is no longer coming from the waffle iron. Remove waffles with a fork.

6. Top with Fruit & Honey Breakfast Spread (see page 31).

Calories 265
  Calories from Fat 100
Total Fat 11.0 g
  Saturated Fat 1.5 g
  Trans Fat 0.0 g
Cholesterol 35 mg
Sodium 435 mg
Potassium 175 mg
Total Carbohydrate 32 g
  Dietary Fiber 1 g
  Sugars 4 g
Protein 8 g
Phosphorus 355 mg

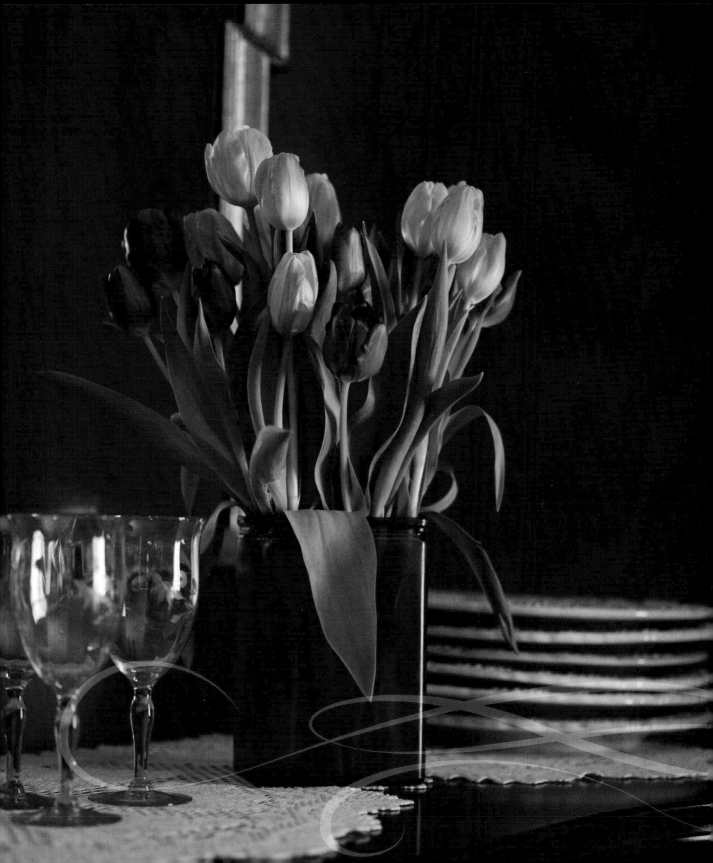

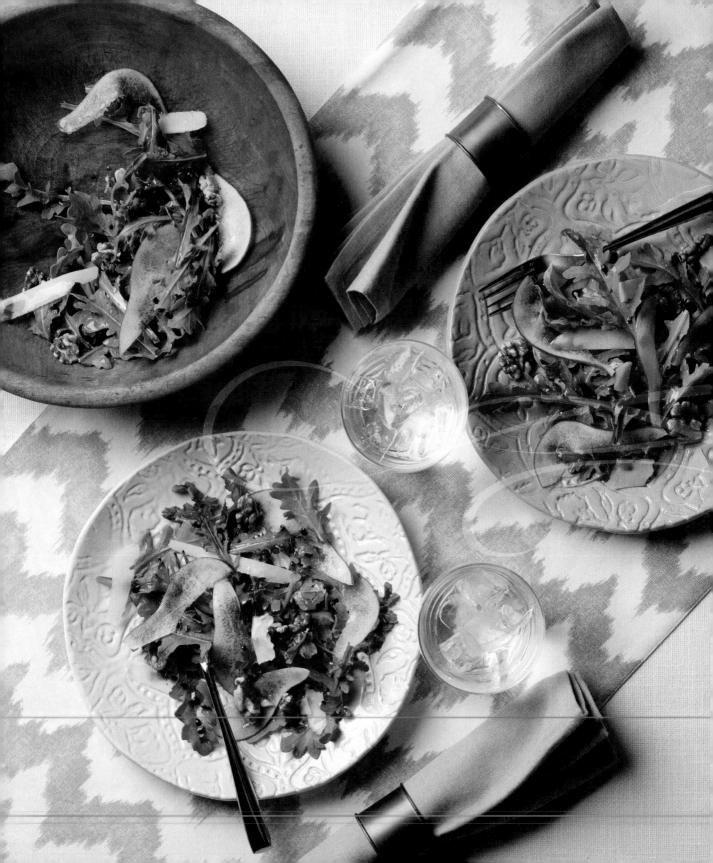

CASUAL ENTERTAINING

Arugula, Pear, Walnut & Pecorino Salad

6 ounces fresh arugula

1 pear

1/4 cup walnut halves

1/4-pound piece of Pecorino Romano, cold (only 1/2 ounce used)

2 tablespoons balsamic vinegar

2 tablespoons extra virgin olive oil

1/2 teaspoon black pepper

Very simple yet beautiful, this is a classic salad in the south of Italy.

SERVES 6 | SERVING SIZE 1/6 recipe | EXCHANGES 1/2 Carbohydrate, 1 1/2 Fat

1. Place the arugula in a large salad bowl. Slice the pear as thinly as possible and place on top of the arugula. Sprinkle with walnut halves. Using a vegetable peeler, shave 1/2 ounce of the Pecorino over the salad bowl.

2. Sprinkle balsamic vinegar over the salad. Sprinkle extra virgin olive oil over the salad. Add pepper. Toss well. Serve.

Calories 105
Calories from Fat 70
Total Fat 8.0 g
Saturated Fat 1.5 g
Trans Fat 0.0 g
Cholesterol 0 mg
Sodium 55 mg
Potassium 165 mg
Total Carbohydrate 7 g
Dietary Fiber 2 g
Sugars 4 g
Protein 2 g
Phosphorus 50 mg

Avocado, Corn & Cherry Tomato Salad

1 pint cherry tomatoes, cut in half

1/2 teaspoon fine sea salt

4–6 thin scallions, sliced 1/2-inch thick on the diagonal

1 cup fresh corn kernels, from an ear of corn, steamed

1 avocado, diced

1/4 cup red wine vinegar

1/4 cup extra virgin olive oil

1/2 cup cilantro or Italian parsley leaves

1/2 to 1 teaspoon ground black pepper

This would be a great salad to serve with a quesadilla, burrito, or chili.

SERVES 8 | SERVING SIZE 1/2 cup | EXCHANGES 1 Vegetable, 2 Fat

1. Place tomatoes in large bowl and sprinkle with salt. Let stand at least 20 minutes.

2. Add scallions, corn, and avocado. Drizzle with vinegar and extra virgin olive oil. Toss. Let stand until serving time.

3. Add cilantro. Season with black pepper and serve.

Calories 120
  Calories from Fat 90
Total Fat 10.0 g
  Saturated Fat 1.4 g
  Trans Fat 0.0 g
Cholesterol 0 mg
Sodium 155 mg
Potassium 270 mg
Total Carbohydrate 8 g
  Dietary Fiber 3 g
  Sugars 2 g
Protein 2 g
Phosphorus 40 mg

Enchilada Casserole

1 teaspoon canola oil

1 pound ground turkey (7% fat)

1 cup sliced scallions (about 1 bunch)

1 medium red bell pepper, chopped (about 1 1/4 cups)

2 cups black beans, drained and rinsed

1 teaspoon no-salt garlic blend seasoning

20 ounces diced tomatoes and green chilies (2 cans Rotel)

1 cup chopped cilantro

5 café-style tortillas made with corn flour (I used Chi Chi brand)

1/2 cup low-fat cheddar cheese (I used Sargento)

This is a great dish to make for a very casual evening in with family. It is easy to prepare and the kids might even enjoy helping!

SERVES 6 | **SERVING SIZE** 3-inch square
EXCHANGES 2 1/2 Starch, 1 Vegetable, 2 Lean Meat, 1 Fat

1. Place canola oil in large sauté pan. Add turkey and sauté until cooked through. Add scallions and bell pepper and sauté until vegetables begin to soften, about 3 minutes. Add black beans, garlic seasoning, and tomatoes and green chilies. Bring to boil, reduce heat to low, and simmer about 10 minutes. Remove from heat and stir in cilantro.

2. Preheat oven to 350°F.

3. Spray a 6 × 9-inch casserole dish with nonstick cooking spray.

4. Place 3 tortillas in the bottom of the pan, cutting them to fit. Spread 3 cups of the mixture on top of the tortillas. Sprinkle with 1/4 cup cheese. Repeat.

5. Bake 20–30 minutes until hot and bubbly. Serve.

Calories 360
  Calories from Fat 100
Total Fat 11.0 g
  Saturated Fat 3.1 g
  Trans Fat 0.1 g
Cholesterol 65 mg
Sodium 590 mg
Potassium 680 mg
Total Carbohydrate 42 g
  Dietary Fiber 9 g
  Sugars 6 g
Protein 27 g
Phosphorus 455 mg

Farro Soup with Mushrooms & Kale

2 tablespoons extra virgin olive oil

1 cup diced onion, or 1/2 of a large onion

1 cup sliced carrots (about 2–3)

1 cup sliced celery (about 2–3 ribs)

2 cups (8 ounces) sliced mushroom

2 cups (12 ounces) uncooked farro

1 teaspoon no-salt garlic seasoning blend

1/2 teaspoon Salt & Pepper Blend (see page viii)

32 ounces low-sodium vegetable stock

6 cups water

8 cups chopped kale, about 1/2 pound

Crushed red pepper (optional)

Cheese rinds (optional)

Farro is a grain often mistaken for wheat, but it is actually a descendent of emmer. It is an ancient grain now grown in Italy with a high fiber content and it is low in gluten. It has a lot of crunch and performs a lot like arborio rice in risotto but retains its distinct crunch. It is rich in fiber, magnesium, and Vitamins A, B, C, and E.

SERVES 10 | **SERVING SIZE** 1 cup | **EXCHANGES** 1 1/2 Starch, 1 Vegetable, 1/2 Fat

1. Place olive oil in large soup pot. Add onion and cook until edges begin to brown. Add carrots, celery, and mushrooms and sauté vegetables 3–4 minutes for added flavor and color.

2. Add farro and mix well with vegetables. Add garlic seasoning and salt and pepper blend. Mix well.

3. Add stock and water. Bring to boil and then reduce to simmer. Cook 20 minutes. Add kale and cook an additional 5–10 minutes to tenderize kale. Add crushed red pepper and cheese rinds (if desired). Serve.

Cook's Tips

ADDING THE LEFTOVER RIND OF A PIECE OF A PARMIGIANO-REGGIANO OR GRANA PADANO WILL ADD A LOT OF FLAVOR WITHOUT A LOT OF CALORIES. THE CRUSHED RED PEPPER WILL PROVIDE A LITTLE KICK TO THE SAVORY GRAINS AND KALE.

Calories 160
  Calories from Fat 35
Total Fat 4.0 g
  Saturated Fat 0.6 g
  Trans Fat 0.0 g
Cholesterol 0 mg
Sodium 175 mg
Potassium 460 mg
Total Carbohydrate 29 g
  Dietary Fiber 8 g
  Sugars 5 g
Protein 7 g
Phosphorus 185 mg

Fresh Tomato and Basil Salad

12 plum tomatoes, roughly chopped

2 cloves garlic, chopped

1 shallot, minced

2 tablespoons extra virgin olive oil

1/2 teaspoon fine sea salt

1/4 teaspoon freshly ground pepper

Splash of red wine vinegar (optional)

1 cup fresh basil leaves

I always make this salad early in the day so that the tomatoes exude all their wonderful juices and the flavors will blend. In summer, I use whatever tomatoes are available at the farmer's market and I will mix different varieties for flavor and texture contrast. But in the off-season, I use plum or Roma tomatoes, as they are always available.

SERVES 4 | SERVING SIZE 1 cup | EXCHANGES 2 Vegetable, 1 Fat

1. Mix tomatoes, garlic, and shallot. Add olive oil, salt, and pepper. Taste for seasoning, and add vinegar, if desired.

2. Tear basil leaves and add to tomato mixture. Serve at room temperature.

VARIATIONS:
- ADD CHUNKS OF FRESH MOZZARELLA.
- ADD 1 SMALL SAUTÉED ZUCCHINI.
- ADD A SLICED CUCUMBER.
- CAN ALSO BE USED AS A TOPPING FOR BRUSCHETTA OR PASTA.

Cook's Tips

FOR BRUSCHETTA: SLICE A LOAF OF GOOD ITALIAN BREAD. GRILL OR BROIL UNTIL BROWNED AND THEN BRUSH WITH EXTRA VIRGIN OLIVE OIL AND RUB WITH A CUT CLOVE OF GARLIC.

Calories 100
Calories from Fat 65
Total Fat 7.0 g
Saturated Fat 1.0 g
Trans Fat 0.0 g
Cholesterol 0 mg
Sodium 305 mg
Potassium 505 mg
Total Carbohydrate 9 g
Dietary Fiber 3 g
Sugars 5 g
Protein 2 g
Phosphorus 55 mg

Italian Fish Soup

2 tablespoons extra virgin olive oil

1 cup diced onion (about 1 medium)

1 cup sliced celery (about 2–3 ribs)

1 cup sliced carrot (about 2–3 carrots)

2 cups (12 ounces) diced Yukon gold potatoes, unpeeled

3 cloves garlic, minced

1 cup fresh basil, chopped

1/2 cup fresh oregano, roughly chopped

1 teaspoon Salt & Pepper Blend (see page viii)

28 ounces canned diced tomatoes

1 green bell pepper, diced

1/4 cup Worcestershire sauce

1 pound fish fillet, such as tilapia, flounder, or cod

48 ounces fish stock or 24 ounces chicken stock with water added (to equal 48 ounces)

A few drops of dry sherry (optional)

Inspired by a soup in Bermuda that was so wonderful, I had to come home and try to recreate it—with an Italian twist.

SERVES 8 | SERVING SIZE 1 1/2 cups | EXCHANGES 1/2 Starch, 2 Vegetable, 2 Lean Meat

1. Place olive oil in the bottom of soup pot. Add the onion, celery, carrot, and potato. Cook on medium heat 5 minutes, stirring occasionally to prevent sticking.

2. Add garlic, basil, oregano, salt, and pepper. Give a quick stir to heat and release aromas of herbs. Cook 1 minute.

3. Add tomatoes, bell pepper, Worcestershire, fish, and fish stock. Simmer 10–15 minutes. Season with salt and pepper to taste.

Cook's Tips

SOUP CAN BE FINISHED WITH A SPLASH OF SHERRY, WHICH GUESTS CAN ADD AS DESIRED.

Calories 180
  Calories from Fat 45
Total Fat 5.0 g
  Saturated Fat 0.9 g
  Trans Fat 0.0 g
Cholesterol 25 mg
Sodium 515 mg
Potassium 840 mg
Total Carbohydrate 20 g
  Dietary Fiber 4 g
  Sugars 6 g
Protein 15 g
Phosphorus 170 mg

Italian Wedding Soup

MEATBALLS

1 large garlic clove, minced

1 large egg

1 small onion, grated (about 1/3 cup)

1 tablespoon chopped fresh basil

1 tablespoon chopped fresh parsley

1/4 cup freshly grated Grana Padano cheese

1/2 teaspoon Salt and Pepper Blend (see page viii)

1/2 cup Italian-style breadcrumbs

1/4 cup low-sodium chicken broth

1 1/4 pounds ground turkey breast

SOUP

1 tablespoon extra virgin olive oil

1 cup sliced carrots (about 3)

1 cup sliced celery (about 3 ribs)

1 cup chopped onion (about 1 medium)

3 quarts low-sodium chicken stock

1 cup uncooked orzo (rice-shaped) pasta

9 ounces baby spinach

Freshly grated Parmigiano-Reggiano (optional)

Calories 200
  Calories from Fat 35
Total Fat 4.0 g
  Saturated Fat 1.3 g
  Trans Fat 0.0 g
Cholesterol 50 mg
Sodium 300 mg
Potassium 595 mg
Total Carbohydrate 21 g
  Dietary Fiber 2 g
  Sugars 3 g
Protein 20 g
Phosphorus 225 mg

Many people think that this soup is served at Italian weddings when, in fact it is called Italian Wedding Soup because the ingredients "marry" so well.

SERVES 12 | **SERVING SIZE** 1 1/3 cups soup (5 meatballs)
EXCHANGES 1 Starch, 1 Vegetable, 2 Lean Meat

1. Mix all meatball ingredients together except turkey. Add turkey and gently mix. Roll into 1–inch meatballs. Try not to overmix or the mixture will be tough. Place meatballs on a parchment–lined baking sheet.

2. Preheat oven to 400°F convection or 425°F traditional bake. Bake 15 minutes and prepare the rest of the soup while meatballs are baking.

3. Place olive oil in 8-quart soup pot. Add carrots, celery, and onion and sauté until onion begins to appear translucent. Add the stock. Bring to a boil and add orzo. Cook 5 minutes. Reduce heat, add meatballs and spinach, and simmer another 10–15 minutes until orzo is completely cooked. Sprinkle with Parmigiano–Reggiano, if desired.

Cook's Tips

USE A 1–INCH ICE CREAM SCOOP TO MAKE FORMING THE MEATBALLS EASIER AND MORE UNIFORM.

A PARMIGIANO RIND IN THE BROTH WOULD ADD GREAT FLAVOR WITH VERY FEW CALORIES.

Lentil Soup with Roasted Garlic & Sun-Dried Tomatoes

2 tablespoons extra virgin olive oil

1 cup chopped onion (about 1 medium)

1 cup sliced carrot (about 3)

1 cup sliced celery, about 3 ribs

1 cup sun-dried tomatoes (not in oil)

1 head roasted garlic (see page 170)

1 pound lentils (I used Umbrian Lentils that are smaller than average green)

1 teaspoon Salt & Pepper Blend (see page viii)

3 quarts chicken or vegetable stock

I love lentil soup, especially when you find small lentils, such as those from Italy or France. These hold up a little better than the average green lentils because they stay firm.

SERVES 12 | **SERVING SIZE** 1 cup | **EXCHANGES** 1 1/2 Starch, 1 Vegetable, 1 Lean Meat

1. Place olive oil in 8-quart soup pot. Add onion, carrots, celery, and sauté 5 minutes. Add sun-dried tomatoes, garlic, lentils, Salt & Pepper Blend, and stock. Bring to a boil. Reduce heat to low and simmer 30 minutes.

Calories 190
  Calories from Fat 25
Total Fat 3.0 g
  Saturated Fat 0.4 g
  Trans Fat 0.0 g
Cholesterol 0 mg
Sodium 365 mg
Potassium 810 mg
Total Carbohydrate 28 g
  Dietary Fiber 9 g
  Sugars 6 g
Protein 15 g
Phosphorus 245 mg

Mango Chicken Salad with Jicama

2 chicken breasts (16 ounces total), poached, cooled, and diced, or equivalent leftover roast or grilled chicken

1/4 cup finely minced red onion

1 large mango, diced into 1/4-inch pieces

1/2 cup jicama, diced into 1/4-inch pieces

1 cup roughly chopped cilantro

1 lime, juiced

6 ounces plain, low-fat Greek yogurt

3 cups chicken stock

Fine sea salt, to taste

Freshly ground pepper, to taste

4 cups mixed greens, washed and dried

1/2 cup toasted sunflower seeds, pumpkin seeds, or soy nuts for garnish

This refreshing salad has a surprise crunch from the diced jicama. The mango adds its own heavenly sweetness and lots of vitamin C.

SERVES 4 | **SERVING SIZE** 1 cup | **EXCHANGES** 1 Fruit, 1 Vegetable, 4 Lean Meat, 1 Fat

1. Mix chicken, red onion, mango, jicama, cilantro, lime juice, and yogurt. Blend well. Add additional yogurt, if necessary, for desired consistency. Add salt and pepper to taste.

2. Serve over mixed greens and garnish with additional mango, seeds, and cilantro.

Cook's Tips

THIS DISH ALSO MAKES A LOVELY HORS D'OEUVRE IF PLACED IN PHYLLO TART SHELLS, WHICH CAN BE PURCHASED AT YOUR SUPERMARKET.

Calories 320
  Calories from Fat 110
Total Fat 12.0 g
  Saturated Fat 2.1 g
  Trans Fat 0.0 g
Cholesterol 65 mg
Sodium 85 mg
Potassium 630 mg
Total Carbohydrate 22 g
  Dietary Fiber 5 g
  Sugars 14 g
Protein 33 g
Phosphorus 410 mg

Mixed Bean Soup

2 tablespoons extra virgin olive oil

1 cup chopped onion (about 1 medium)

1 cup sliced celery (about 3 ribs)

1 cup sliced carrots (about 3)

3 cloves garlic, minced

15 ounces small white beans, drained and rinsed

15 ounces canned pink beans, drained and rinsed

15 ounces black beans, drained and rinsed

28 ounces canned diced tomatoes

3 bay leaves

1 cup fresh basil leaves, chopped

1/2 cup fresh oregano, chopped

32 ounces unsalted vegetable stock

I love preparing a big pot of soup and inviting neighbors in on a cold day for a seat by the fire with a nice soup, salad, and glass of wine. This soup would also be delicious with the Enchilada Casserole (page 50) or the Avocado, Corn, and Cherry Tomato Salad (page 49).

SERVES 8 | **SERVING SIZE** 2 cups | **EXCHANGES** 1 1/2 Starch, 2 Vegetable, 1 Lean Meat

1. Put olive oil in 8–quart stockpot. Add onion, celery, carrots, and garlic. Cook until garlic is fragrant and onion becomes translucent.

2. Add beans, tomatoes, bay leaves, basil, oregano, and stock. Simmer 20–30 minutes.

3. Garnish with fresh herbs. Remove bay leaves before serving.

Calories 205
Calories from Fat 40
Total Fat 4.5 g
Saturated Fat 0.6 g
Trans Fat 0.0 g
Cholesterol 0 mg
Sodium 445 mg
Potassium 745 mg
Total Carbohydrate 34 g
Dietary Fiber 11 g
Sugars 6 g
Protein 9 g
Phosphorus 180 mg

Mushroom Onion Soup

20 ounces mushrooms, such as portobello or cremini

1 tablespoon extra virgin olive oil

1 tablespoon sweet butter

2 large sweet onions, thinly sliced

4 cloves garlic, minced

32 ounces fat-free, low-sodium mushroom, chicken, or vegetable stock

Fresh chopped herbs, for garnish

This recipe combines two favorite soups that both have very few calories. A sprinkle of cheese would be lovely if your meal plan will allow.

SERVES 8 | SERVING SIZE 1 cup | **EXCHANGES** 2 Vegetable, 1/2 Fat

1. Slice or chop mushrooms into bite–sized pieces.

2. Thinly film pan with olive oil and add butter. Melt butter in oil and add onion. Cook until onions are translucent. Add garlic and cook until fragrant.

3. Add mushrooms to pan. Cook 3–5 minutes until moisture is released. Add stock and cook 30 minutes.

4. Purée mixture with stick blender but leave some pieces of mushroom. Garnish with fresh herbs and serve.

Calories 80
Calories from Fat 30
Total Fat 3.5 g
Saturated Fat 1.2 g
Trans Fat 0.1 g
Cholesterol 5 mg
Sodium 280 mg
Potassium 495 mg
Total Carbohydrate 10 g
Dietary Fiber 1 g
Sugars 6 g
Protein 4 g
Phosphorus 125 mg

Pork & Sweet Potato Stew

2 pounds boneless country pork ribs

1/4 cup Wondra flour

1 teaspoon Salt & Pepper Blend (page viii)

1 tablespoon canola oil

1 pound sweet potatoes, cut into 2-inch cubes (about 2 cups)

1 large onion, chopped (about 1 cup)

2 large cloves garlic, crushed with the side of a knife and peeled

3 medium carrots, ends trimmed, scrubbed, and cut into 2-inch lengths (about 1 cup)

3 celery stalks, ends trimmed, scrubbed and cut into 2-inch lengths (about 1 cup)

1 tablespoon dry Italian seasoning blend

1 quart low-sodium vegetable stock

1/2 cup dry red wine

1 medium zucchini, sliced about 1/2 inch thick (about 1 cup)

This one-pot comfort meal is reminiscent of something grandma would have made, with the added nutritional punch from the sweet potato and all the vegetables. Prepare this a day or two ahead of serving and transfer to your crockpot or slow cooker and cook for 4 hours on high or 8 hours on low.

SERVES 10 | **SERVING SIZE** 1 cup | **EXCHANGES** 1/2 Starch, 1 Vegetable, 2 Lean Meat, 1 Fat

1. Cut pork into bite-sized pieces. Mix Wondra and salt and pepper blend together in a large bowl. Add pork and coat evenly. You will have about 1 tablespoon flour mixture left. Mix with 1/4 cup water and reserve for sauce. Set aside in refrigerator.

2. Place canola oil in 6-quart stockpot. Heat pan to medium. (Test pan for proper heat by touching a piece of pork to the pan. If you hear a sizzle, it's ready.) Place the meat in a single layer. Sear the meat until nicely browned on all sides. Remove from pan and set aside while sautéing vegetables.

3. Add potatoes, onion, garlic, carrots, celery, and Italian seasoning. Sauté 3–5 minutes until vegetables begin to brown and seasoning becomes fragrant. Return pork to pan.

4. Add stock, wine, and reserved flour and water mixture. Stir. Bring to boil for 2 minutes. Reduce heat to low and cook 30 minutes. Add zucchini and cook an additional 30 minutes. Serve.

Calories 205
Calories from Fat 70
Total Fat 8.0 g
Saturated Fat 2.5 g
Trans Fat 0.0 g
Cholesterol 55 mg
Sodium 290 mg
Potassium 620 mg
Total Carbohydrate 16 g
Dietary Fiber 3 g
Sugars 6 g
Protein 18 g
Phosphorus 235 mg

Roasted Beet Salad

2 pounds fresh beets, weighed
    without tops (about 4 cups cut up)

2 teaspoons extra virgin olive oil

1/2 teaspoon fine sea salt

2 tablespoons balsamic vinegar

Beets have gotten a bad rap because of poor processing, but when you purchase fresh beets and roast them, they are a sweet treat. They are delicious with a balsamic drizzle. I get very excited when I see baby beets in different colors in the market and can create a beautiful as well as tasty dish.

SERVES 6 | SERVING SIZE 2/3 cup | EXCHANGES 2 Vegetable

1. Peel beets and cut them into quarters or eighths, depending on how large they are. I like them a little larger than bite-sized. If baby beets are available, do not cut them.

2. Toss with extra virgin olive oil and salt. Place in foil pan and roast at 425°F for 20–40 minutes, depending on the size of the beets. Begin testing at 20 minutes. They should be fork tender.

3. Place in serving dish and drizzle with balsamic vinegar. Sprinkle some goat cheese on the beets if your meal plan permits.

Calories 60
    Calories from Fat 15
Total Fat 1.5 g
    Saturated Fat 0.2 g
    Trans Fat 0.0 g
Cholesterol 0 mg
Sodium 270 mg
Potassium 295 mg
Total Carbohydrate 10 g
    Dietary Fiber 2 g
    Sugars 8 g
Protein 2 g
Phosphorus 35 mg

Roasted Pepper Salad with Extra Virgin Olive Oil

4 roasted peppers in a variety of colors (see Roasted Peppers, page 20), peeled and cut into quarters

1/2 teaspoon fine sea salt

Freshly ground black pepper, to taste

3 cloves garlic, minced

2 tablespoons extra virgin olive oil

Edible flowers (such as nasturtiums), for garnish (optional)

I always include a salad with every meal and this particular one will give some variety to your salad repertoire. It is also great as part of an Al Fresco or Italian menu. If you are able to get four colors of peppers, you can serve each person one quarter of each pepper in all the colors for a visually and nutritionally appealing salad.

SERVES 4 | **SERVING SIZE** 1 pepper | **EXCHANGES** 2 Vegetable, 1 Fat

1. Place peppers on platter. Sprinkle with salt, freshly ground black pepper, and minced garlic. Drizzle with good-quality extra virgin olive oil. Garnish platter with edible flowers such as nasturtiums.

Cook's Tips

CAN BE MADE A DAY IN ADVANCE TO ALLOW FLAVORS TO BLEND.

Calories 100
Calories from Fat 65
Total Fat 7.0 g
Saturated Fat 1.0 g
Trans Fat 0.0 g
Cholesterol 0 mg
Sodium 300 mg
Potassium 300 mg
Total Carbohydrate 9 g
Dietary Fiber 2 g
Sugars 5 g
Protein 1 g
Phosphorus 35 mg

Shaved Brussels Sprouts Salad with Walnuts & Pecorino Cheese

2 cups fresh Brussels sprouts

1 medium red onion

1/2 cup chopped walnuts

1/4 cup grated Pecorino Romano cheese

1 1/2 tablespoons orange-infused extra virgin olive oil

1 tablespoon white wine vinegar

1/2 teaspoon fine sea salt

1/2 teaspoon freshly ground black pepper

Brussels sprouts are often maligned, but when you have them properly prepared, they are surprisingly delicious!

SERVES 8 | **SERVING SIZE** 1/2 cup | **EXCHANGES** 1 Vegetable, 1 1/2 Fat

1. Wash and trim the Brussels sprouts. Place in food processor fitted with slicing disk. Slice the Brussels sprouts and place in large salad bowl. Repeat with red onion. Combine onion and Brussels sprouts.

2. Add remaining ingredients to salad bowl. Mix well.

Cook's Tips

CAN BE MADE EARLY IN THE DAY AND REFRIGERATED UNTIL SERVING TIME.

Calories 100
Calories from Fat 70
Total Fat 8.0 g
Saturated Fat 1.4 g
Trans Fat 0.0 g
Cholesterol 0 mg
Sodium 200 mg
Potassium 150 mg
Total Carbohydrate 5 g
Dietary Fiber 2 g
Sugars 1 g
Protein 3 g
Phosphorus 65 mg

Thai Chicken Chili

2 tablespoons canola oil

1 cup chopped onion (about 1 medium)

1 cup sliced carrot (about 3)

1 cup sliced celery (about 3 ribs)

2 garlic cloves, minced

1 3/4 pounds boneless, skinless chicken breast, cut into bite-sized cubes (about 4 cups)

2 tablespoons sweet ginger garlic seasoning (I used Simply Asia brand)

2 cups cannellini beans, drained and rinsed well

1 cup chopped red bell pepper (about 1 medium)

10 ounces whole water chestnuts, halved

1/4 cup cream of coconut

2 cups low-sodium chicken stock

I love all the wonderful Thai spiciness that this cuisine brings to the table. Recently, I attended a food showcase and was given a sample of a delicious seasoning blend called sweet ginger garlic that was the inspiration for this dish.

SERVES 8 | **SERVING SIZE** 1 cup | **EXCHANGES** 1/2 Starch, 2 Vegetable, 3 Lean Meat, 1 Fat

1. Place canola oil in 8-quart stockpot. Add onion, carrots, celery, garlic, and chicken and cook until chicken is browned, about 7 minutes.

2. Push this mixture to the side and add seasoning blend. Toast for 1–2 minutes until fragrant.

3. Add beans, bell pepper, water chestnuts, coconut, and chicken stock and mix well. Bring to a boil and immediately reduce heat to a simmer. Cook 30 minutes or longer.

4. Serve with rice or a small grain, such as quinoa.

Calories 275
Calories from Fat 70
Total Fat 8.0 g
Saturated Fat 2.6 g
Trans Fat 0.0 g
Cholesterol 60 mg
Sodium 370 mg
Potassium 665 mg
Total Carbohydrate 22 g
Dietary Fiber 6 g
Sugars 5 g
Protein 27 g
Phosphorus 265 mg

Tre Colore Salad with Pomegranate & Cinnamon Spiced Walnuts with Balsamic Vinaigrette

1 head green leaf lettuce

1 small head radicchio

1 medium head Belgian endive

1/2 pomegranate, seeded

1/2 cup pomegranate seeds

1/4 cup Cinnamon Spiced Walnuts (see page 162)

1 tablespoon crumbled Gorgonzola cheese

4 tablespoons Basic Vinaigrette (page 173)

This quick, healthy salad is so beautiful and tasty you will want to serve it to your guests at every meal! The Basic Vinaigrette can be used as a salad dressing or as a marinade.

SERVES 6 | SERVING SIZE 1/6 recipe | EXCHANGES 1/2 Carbohydrate, 2 Fat

1. Wash and dry lettuce, radicchio, and endive. Place in large salad bowl. Add pomegranate, pomegranate seeds, and nuts. Sprinkle with cheese. Drizzle with Basic Vinaigrette (page 173).

VARIATIONS:
- USE DIFFERENT TYPES AND FLAVORS OF VINEGAR
- ADD 1–2 DROPS ORANGE OIL OR ORANGE EXTRACT
- TRY ADDING CHOPPED FRESH HERBS, ROASTED GARLIC, FRESH RASPBERRIES, OR CRUSHED CRANBERRIES.
- FRENCH VINAIGRETTE: ADD 1 TEASPOON DIJON MUSTARD

Cook's Tips

SLOWLY WHISKING IN THE OIL ALLOWS FOR A BETTER EMULSION.

Calories 115
  Calories from Fat 80
Total Fat 9.0 g
  Saturated Fat 1.4 g
  Trans Fat 0.0 g
Cholesterol 0 mg
Sodium 60 mg
Potassium 245 mg
Total Carbohydrate 7 g
  Dietary Fiber 2 g
  Sugars 3 g
Protein 2 g
Phosphorus 50 mg

Chicken Waldorf Salad

8 ounces boneless, skinless chicken breast

1 Granny Smith apple (about 2 cups), chopped

1 lemon, juiced (about 1/4 cup)

1/2 cup pomegranate arils (seeds)

1/2 cup walnuts

1/2 teaspoon Salt & Pepper Blend (page viii)

1/2 cup plain, nonfat yogurt

1 tablespoon honey

SERVES 4 | SERVING SIZE 1 cup
EXCHANGES 1 Fruit, 1/2 Carbohydrate, 2 Lean Meat, 1 1/2 Fat

1. Place chicken breast in sauté pan and cover with water. Bring to boil and immediately turn down to low. Cook 9–10 minutes. Turn heat off. Let sit 10–20 minutes to cool in the cooking liquid. Drain and chop into bite–sized pieces.

2. While chicken is cooking and cooling, chop apple. Place apple in large bowl with lemon juice. Add pomegranate, walnuts, Salt & Pepper Blend, yogurt, and honey. Mix well. Add chicken and mix again. Chill until serving time.

Calories 230
  Calories from Fat 100
Total Fat 11.0 g
  Saturated Fat 1.3 g
  Trans Fat 0.0 g
Cholesterol 30 mg
Sodium 240 mg
Potassium 325 mg
Total Carbohydrate 21 g
  Dietary Fiber 3 g
  Sugars 15 g
Protein 14 g
Phosphorus 175 mg

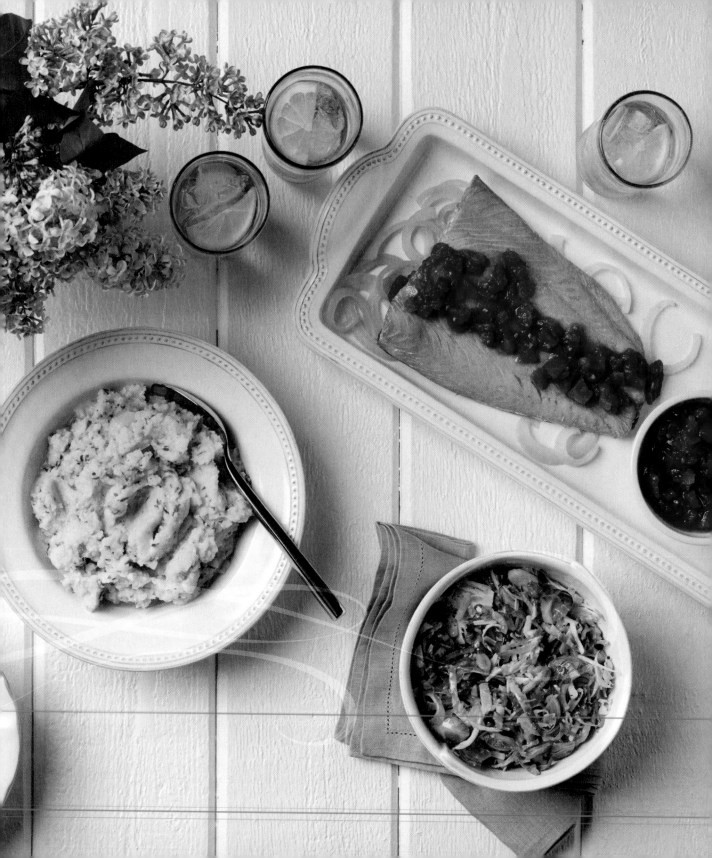

DAZZLING
DINNER PARTIES

Brisket with Red Wine Reduction

2 tablespoons extra virgin olive oil

1 beef brisket (about 3 pounds)

3 large cloves garlic, chopped

1 large onion, chopped

1 teaspoon fine sea salt

1 teaspoon coarse ground black pepper

1 1/2 cups dry red wine, such as Pinot Noir, Chianti, or Syrah; or beef broth; or a combination of wine and broth

10 ounces cremini mushroooms, quartered

1 tablespoon Wondra flour

This dish can be made a day or two ahead and serves a crowd. The longer cooking time of this recipe is necessary for a tender brisket, but it also causes the meat to shrink. This dish can be turned into a one-pot meal by adding some carrots and potatoes. Serve with a Tre Colore salad (page 64).

SERVES 8 | SERVING SIZE 1/8 recipe | EXCHANGES 1 Vegetable, 4 Lean Meat, 1 1/2 Fat

1. Preheat oven to 275°F.

2. Place extra virgin olive oil in the bottom of the braising or sauté pan. Heat to medium high and add brisket. Cook until the brisket is nicely browned. Turn and brown on other side. While second side is browning, place garlic and onions in pan around brisket. Sprinkle salt and pepper over brisket and rub it in. (You can also add some fresh herbs if you have them. A sprig of rosemary is nice.)

3. Once onions begin to brown, add wine or broth. (It will deglaze pan and lift all the good stuff off the bottom of the pan.) Add mushrooms, cover, and place in preheated oven for 2–3 hours until fork tender. If possible, cool in the same pan. Once cooled, remove brisket to cutting board. Bring the pan juices to a boil and reduce until thickened. You can also add a sprinkle or two of Wondra flour to help thicken. Pour the sauce over the brisket and reheat covered, if desired.

Calories 270
   Calories from Fat 115
Total Fat 13.0 g
   Saturated Fat 4.1 g
   Trans Fat 0.0 g
Cholesterol 90 mg
Sodium 370 mg
Potassium 495 mg
Total Carbohydrate 5 g
   Dietary Fiber 1 g
   Sugars 2 g
Protein 31 g
Phosphorus 295 mg

Fresh Herb Cauliflower

1 head cauliflower, washed and broken into florets

1 teaspoon Salt & Pepper Blend (page viii)

1 tablespoon trans-fat–free tub margarine

1/2 cup freshly chopped Italian parsley

When you don't want to have a standard side dish like mashed potatoes or any other starch, you can serve this "mashed" cauliflower and your guests will be surprised and satisfied with fewer calories. For a lovely presentation, you can place a serving of the Cauliflower inside of a radicchio leaf.

SERVES 4 | **SERVING SIZE** 1/4 recipe | **EXCHANGES** 1 Vegetable, 1/2 Fat

1. Place the cauliflower and Salt & Pepper Blend in a 6–8 quart saucepan and cover with water. Cover and bring to a boil. Cook until cauliflower is fork tender, about 10 minutes.

2. Drain and place in large bowl or mixer bowl. Add margarine and mash cauliflower until smooth. You can use a hand mixer or stand mixer. Stir in parsley and serve in place of mashed potatoes.

Calories 40
Calories from Fat 20
Total Fat 2.5 g
Saturated Fat 0.7 g
Trans Fat 0.0 g
Cholesterol 0 mg
Sodium 425 mg
Potassium 140 mg
Total Carbohydrate 4 g
Dietary Fiber 2 g
Sugars 2 g
Protein 2 g
Phosphorus 30 mg

Cedar Plank Salmon with Irish Whiskey Sauce

Cedar plank (food grade, purchase at grocery or gourmet store)

2 teaspoons canola oil

1 cup chopped onion (about 1 large)

2 cloves garlic, peeled and minced

15 ounces petite, diced tomatoes

1 cup low-sodium chicken stock

1 tablespoon Worcestershire sauce

1/4 cup Irish whiskey

1/4 teaspoon freshly ground black pepper

1 large onion, sliced 1/4 inch thick

1 pound salmon fillet, with skin

SERVES 4 | SERVING SIZE 1/4 recipe | **EXCHANGES** 3 Vegetable, 3 Lean Meat, 2 Fat

1. Preheat oven to 400°F.

2. Soak cedar plank in water for at least 20 minutes while preparing whiskey sauce. This will prevent charring.

3. Place canola oil in saucepan. Add chopped onion and cook until it begins to brown. Add garlic and cook until garlic becomes fragrant, about 1 minute. Add tomatoes, stock, Worcestershire sauce, whiskey, and pepper. Bring to a boil, reduce heat, and simmer 20 minutes.

4. In the meantime, remove cedar plank from water and place on large baking sheet. Spread sliced onion on plank. Place salmon fillet, skin side down, on top of onions. Brush top of salmon lightly with 2 tablespoons of the whiskey sauce. Bake 25–30 minutes until fish is cooked completely.

5. Serve with cedar plank onions and additional whiskey sauce on the side.

Calories 300
  Calories from Fat 115
Total Fat 13.0 g
  Saturated Fat 2.0 g
  Trans Fat 0.0 g
Cholesterol 80 mg
Sodium 280 mg
Potassium 775 mg
Total Carbohydrate 15 g
  Dietary Fiber 3 g
  Sugars 7 g
Protein 28 g
Phosphorus 315 mg

Chicken and Vegetables en Papillote

Parchment paper

24 thin slices of Yukon gold potatoes, about 1 small potato per person

4 pieces boneless, skinless chicken breasts (approximately 4 ounces each)

4 cloves garlic, minced

4 sprigs rosemary

4 sprigs thyme

24 fresh green beans

12 baby carrots, halved lengthwise

1 small yellow squash, cut into 16 julienned pieces

1 teaspoon Salt & Pepper Blend (page viii)

1/2 cup dry white wine, such as Pinot Grigio, Soave, Orvieto, or Sauvignon Blanc

This is a perfect spa dish you can make at home. It is also a dramatic dish to serve to guests. When you place the parchment package on each guest's dinner plate, and when they open it, the steam and the flavors will be intoxicating! Fish fillets also work well in this recipe.

SERVES 4 | SERVING SIZE 1 package | EXCHANGES 2 Starch, 1 Vegetable, 3 Lean Meat

1. Preheat oven to 375°F.

2. Cut 4 sheets of parchment, about 18 inches long, and then fold each in half lengthwise. Cut each into a 1/2 heart shape, which will make a heart when fully opened.

3. Working on 1/2 of the heart, layer as follows: 6 slices potato, chicken breast, garlic, rosemary, thyme, 6 green beans, 6 pieces carrot, and 4 pieces yellow squash.

4. Sprinkle with salt and pepper and wine.

5. Fold the parchment in half and crimp edges all the way around to seal tightly. Place on baking sheet and place in the preheated oven. Bake 25–30 minutes.

~**VARIATIONS:** FOIL CAN BE USED IN PLACE OF PARCHMENT PAPER AND CAN BE COOKED OUTSIDE ON THE GRILL.

Calories 290
  Calories from Fat 25
Total Fat 3.0 g
  Saturated Fat 0.9 g
  Trans Fat 0.0 g
Cholesterol 65 mg
Sodium 480 mg
Potassium 970 mg
Total Carbohydrate 35 g
  Dietary Fiber 5 g
  Sugars 5 g
Protein 28 g
Phosphorus 335 mg

Chicken Breast with Ricotta Salata & Fresh Basil

1/4 cup breadcrumbs

1 1/4 cups dry white wine, such as Orvieto or Pinot Grigio (divided use)

1 ounce ricotta salata, grated

1/2 cup fresh basil, chopped

1/2 cup fresh Italian parsley, chopped

1/2 teaspoon fine sea salt

1/4 teaspoon freshly ground black pepper

4 (5-ounce) boneless chicken breasts, with skin and a pocket for stuffing

2 teaspoons extra virgin olive oil

8 tomato slices

Ricotta salata, also known as dry ricotta, is a delicious smooth, firm sheep's milk cheese that can be grated. It is generally sold in chunks and is imported from Italy.

SERVES 4 | SERVING SIZE 1/4 recipe | EXCHANGES 1/2 Carbohydrate, 4 Lean Meat

1. Soak breadcrumbs in 1/4 cup white wine.

2. Mix grated ricotta salata with basil and parsley and add wine-soaked breadcrumbs. Season with salt and pepper.

3. Stuff each chicken breast with 1/4 of the cheese mixture. Season the outside with salt and pepper.

4. Place olive oil in sauté pan and brown chicken on both sides, skin side first. Turn chicken and add 1 cup wine to deglaze pan. Cover and cook until chicken is done, approximately 10 minutes. Remove skin from chicken before serving. Serve with 2 slices of tomato per serving.

Calories 240
  Calories from Fat 65
Total Fat 7.0 g
  Saturated Fat 2.3 g
  Trans Fat 0.0 g
Cholesterol 80 mg
Sodium 535 mg
Potassium 395 mg
Total Carbohydrate 8 g
  Dietary Fiber 1 g
  Sugars 2 g
Protein 29 g
Phosphorus 235 mg

Duck Breast with Cognac-Soaked Cherries

1 pound magret duck breast

2 tablespoons roasted garlic purée
(see recipe for Roasted Garlic,
page 170)

1/4 teaspoon fine sea salt

1/2 teaspoon freshly ground pepper

1/2 cup brandy

1/2 cup cognac

1/4 cup dried cherries

1 tablespoon extra virgin olive oil

1/4 cup chicken stock

The earlier that you rub this duck with the roasted garlic the better! It is great for a dinner party or a romantic evening.

SERVES 4 | SERVING SIZE 1/4 recipe | EXCHANGES 1 Carbohydrate, 2 Lean Meat, 1/2 Alcohol

1. Trim all visible fat from duck breast. Rub with garlic purée. Season with salt and pepper. Pour brandy into plastic bag. Add duck. Let stand in refrigerator until cooking time.

2. Place cognac in small saucepan. Bring to boil. Add cherries and remove from heat. Let cherries steep in cognac while cooking the duck. (This can also be done earlier in the day.)

3. Drain cognac from cherries. Reserve cognac for sauce. Reserve cherries for finishing the dish.

4. Preheat oven to 400°F at least 15 minutes prior to sautéing the duck.

5. Heat sauté pan. Drain duck and pat dry. Place olive oil in pan large enough to hold the duck breast. Add duck and sear on both sides.

6. Place sauté pan in the center of your oven and roast until your meat thermometer reads 125°F; check for doneness at approximately 10 minutes. Remove from oven and place duck breast on cutting board to rest.

7. Using the same sauté pan, add the drained and reserved cognac and the chicken stock and return pan to medium heat. Heat the cognac/stock mixture on high to deglaze the sauté pan. Cook until the sauce reduces slightly and becomes more syrupy.

8. Slice the duck breast on a diagonal, plate, and pour the cognac over the duck. Garnish with the cherries.

VARIATIONS: RECIPE CAN ALSO BE USED FOR A SHELL STEAK INSTEAD OF DUCK BREAST.

Cook's Tips

THIS DISH IS NICE SERVED WITH A SALAD OF MIXED BABY GREENS WITH A BALSAMIC VINAIGRETTE, WALNUTS, AND CRUMBLED BLUE CHEESE, AND OVEN-ROASTED WHITE AND SWEET POTATOES OR WILD RICE.

Calories 210
  Calories from Fat 45
Total Fat 5.0 g
  Saturated Fat 0.9 g
  Trans Fat 0.0 g
Cholesterol 80 mg
Sodium 370 mg
Potassium 245 mg
Total Carbohydrate 14 g
  Dietary Fiber 1 g
  Sugars 7 g
Protein 16 g
Phosphorus 195 mg

DAZZLING
DINNER
PARTIES

Filet Mignon & Shrimp with Red Wine Reduction

2 pieces filet mignon (about 6 ounces each)

Salt & Pepper Blend (page viii)

Extra virgin olive oil

SAUCE

2 teaspoons extra virgin olive oil

1 large shallot, finely minced

1/2 cup red wine (broth, stock, or water will substitute)

1 cup low-sodium beef, mushroom, or vegetable stock

GARNISH

4 large shrimp, steamed, peeled, and deveined (optional)

A perfect recipe for dinner for two, for Christmas, or any other time.

SERVES 2 | **SERVING SIZE** 1 piece filet mignon | **EXCHANGES** 5 Lean Meat, 2 Fat

1. Take meat out of the refrigerator about 20 minutes before cooking time. Sprinkle Salt & Pepper Blend on both sides of the steaks. Rub with a few drops of extra virgin olive oil.

2. Preheat skillet. Place filet in skillet and cook for 3–5 minutes per side for rare to medium rare. If the outside of the filet is cooking too quickly, you can reduce heat to medium and cover. Test for doneness with a meat thermometer. Rare is 125°F, medium is 140°F. Remove from pan and place on cutting board to rest.

3. In the meantime, add olive oil and shallots to small sauté pan. Cook 1 minute. Add the red wine and reduce until liquid is almost all evaporated. Add stock. Reduce by half and serve over filet mignon.

4. Garnish with steamed shrimp placed on top of the filet in a heart shape or serve the shrimp cocktail as an appetizer, if desired.

Calories 345
Calories from Fat 145
Total Fat 16.0 g
Saturated Fat 4.4 g
Trans Fat 0.0 g
Cholesterol 150 mg
Sodium 475 mg
Potassium 600 mg
Total Carbohydrate 4 g
Dietary Fiber 1 g
Sugars 1 g
Protein 40 g
Phosphorus 365 mg

DAZZLING DINNER PARTIES

Grilled Tuna with White Soybean Salad with Lemon & Thyme

1/2 teaspoon extra virgin olive oil, divided use

8 large cloves garlic, sliced lengthwise

1 lemon, juiced

8 sprigs fresh thyme

8 ounces canned white soybeans, drained and rinsed well

1/2 teaspoon Salt & Pepper Blend (divided use) (page viii)

4 tuna steaks (about 5 ounces each)

SERVES 4 | **SERVING SIZE** 1 tuna steak | **EXCHANGES** 1/2 Starch, 5 Lean Meat, 1 1/2 Fat

1. Place 1/4 teaspoon olive oil in small sauté or saucepan. Add sliced garlic and cook over medium–high heat. Watch carefully and cook until golden. Remove garlic from oil with slotted spoon and place on paper towels. Set aside.

2. Mix the warm olive oil with lemon juice, thyme, and beans. Add 1/4 teaspoon Salt & Pepper Blend. Set aside to allow flavors to blend. This salad can be made a day or two ahead of time.

3. Place tuna on a dinner plate and rub with 1/4 teaspoon extra virgin olive oil and sprinkle with 1/4 teaspoon Salt & Pepper Blend.

4. Place tuna steak on grill and grill to desired doneness.

5. Serve the white soybean salad with grilled tuna and top with toasted garlic chips.

Calories 340
  Calories from Fat 155
Total Fat 17.0 g
  Saturated Fat 3.2 g
  Trans Fat 0.0 g
Cholesterol 55 mg
Sodium 365 mg
Potassium 565 mg
Total Carbohydrate 6 g
  Dietary Fiber 2 g
  Sugars 1 g
Protein 40 g
Phosphorus 455 mg

DAZZLING DINNER PARTIES

Osso Buco in Cremolata*

2 medium carrots, peeled and roughly chopped

1 medium onion, peeled and quartered

1 celery stalk, washed and roughly chopped

4 tablespoons olive oil (divided use)

6 pieces (about 3 pounds) veal shank,-bone-in with marrow

1/2 cup all-purpose flour (for dusting the veal)

1/2 teaspoon Salt & Pepper Blend (page viii)

1 cup dry red wine

2 cups water

CREMOLATA

1 lemon, zested

1/2 cup chopped parsley

1 or 2 cloves garlic, peeled and finely chopped

Osso Buco is truly one of my favorite dishes to eat but also to serve to guests. This is a wonderful do-ahead dish and great with a glass of Barolo wine. Both the dish and the wine are from the Piedmont region of Italy. Traditionally, Osso Buco is served with risotto, but I enjoy it with Celery Root Purée (page 171), which has fewer carbs.

SERVES 4 | SERVING SIZE 1/4 recipe
EXCHANGES 1/2 Starch, 3 Vegetable, 5 Lean Meat, 1 Fat

1. Preheat oven to 350°F.

2. Put the carrots, onion, and celery into food processor and chop until almost minced (or finely chop by hand).

3. Place just enough of the olive oil in a large sauté pan to give a good crust to the veal; add the vegetables and sauté until softened.

4. Dust veal with flour (discard remaining flour). Heat remaining 2 tablespoons of olive oil in large sauté pan and add meat in single layer. Brown on both sides and season with Salt and Pepper Blend. Add the wine and cook until most of the wine has evaporated. Add the vegetables and water. Cover the dish and place in the oven for 1–2 hours until meat is tender.

5. Remove the foil for the last 20–30 minutes of cooking. Add more water if necessary

6. Mix Cremolata ingredients together. Serve with Osso Buco.

Cook's Tips

PAIR FOOD WITH A WINE FROM THE SAME REGION.

Calories 400
Calories from Fat 135
Total Fat 15.0 g
Saturated Fat 3.3 g
Trans Fat 0.0 g
Cholesterol 145 mg
Sodium 555 mg
Potassium 950 mg
Total Carbohydrate 21 g
Dietary Fiber 4 g
Sugars 6 g
Protein 42 g
Phosphorus 380 mg

**DAZZLING
DINNER
PARTIES**

Recipe adapted for the American Kitchen by Barbara Seelig-Brown, courtesy of Chef Luisa from Arte e Cucina Cooking School.

Oven-Roasted Baby Yukon Gold Potatoes

3 pounds baby Yukon gold, red, or fingerling potatoes

1 tablespoon extra virgin olive oil

1 teaspoon fine sea salt

1/2 teaspoon coarsely ground black pepper

1 teaspoon rosemary leaves

SERVES 6 | SERVING SIZE 1/6 recipe | **EXCHANGES** 2 1/2 Starch

1. Preheat oven to 450°F.

2. Wash and dry potatoes. Place in baking dish and toss with olive oil, salt, pepper, and rosemary.

3. Roast about 30 minutes or until tender when a fork is inserted.

Calories 180
  Calories from Fat 20
Total Fat 2.5 g
  Saturated Fat 0.4 g
  Trans Fat 0.0 g
Cholesterol 0 mg
Sodium 405 mg
Potassium 875 mg
Total Carbohydrate 36 g
  Dietary Fiber 5 g
  Sugars 2 g
Protein 4 g
Phosphorus 120 mg

Pork Chops with Vinegar Peppers

4 pork chops (about 5 ounces each), 1 inch thick

1/4 teaspoon Salt & Pepper Blend (page viii)

1 tablespoon extra virgin olive oil

2 cloves garlic, minced

1 cup jarred hot or mild cherry peppers, seeded

1/4 cup juice from peppers

1/4 cup water

This is a classic Southern Italian dish that is so quick and easy it's hard to believe it's so full of flavor. Serve with Fresh Herb Cauliflower (page 69). A nice start to the meal would be the Farro Soup with Mushrooms and Kale (page 51).

SERVES 4 | SERVING SIZE 1/4 recipe | **EXCHANGES** 3 Lean Meat, 1 Fat

1. Sprinkle the chops evenly with Salt & Pepper Blend. Place the olive oil in a large sauté pan. Heat pan to medium–high heat and add chops. Brown on first side and then turn.

2. Scatter garlic around the chops on the pan surface so that it begins to brown. Once the chops are browned on second side, add peppers, pepper juice, and water. Cook 5 minutes and serve.

Calories 180
Calories from Fat 80
Total Fat 9.0 g
Saturated Fat 2.6 g
Trans Fat 0.0 g
Cholesterol 60 mg
Sodium 465 mg
Potassium 340 mg
Total Carbohydrate 1 g
Dietary Fiber 0 g
Sugars 0 g
Protein 21 g
Phosphorus 140 mg

Pork Cutlets with Champagne Mustard & Sautéed Apples

4 boneless pork chops, approximately 1/2 inch thick

3/4 teaspoon Salt & Pepper Blend (page viii)

4 Granny Smith apples

1 lemon, juiced

1/2 teaspoon ground cinnamon

2 tablespoons light brown sugar

Whole nutmeg

4 teaspoons olive oil (divided use)

1/2 cup cider or apple juice

1/4 cup Champagne mustard

1 clove garlic, minced

1 small onion, finely chopped

1/2–1 cup dry white wine

2 teaspoons beef broth or concentrated broth

1 teaspoon Worcestershire sauce

This is a nice dish to prepare in the fall when apples are crisp and juicy.

SERVES 4 | SERVING SIZE 1/4 recipe
EXCHANGES 1 1/2 Fruit, 1/2 Carbohydrate, 3 Lean Meat, 1 1/2 Fat

1. Season both sides of pork with salt and pepper. Set aside.

2. Slice apples 1/4 inch thick and sprinkle with lemon juice to delay browning. Season with cinnamon, sugar, and a fresh grinding of nutmeg.

3. Thinly film one sauté pan with 2 teaspoons olive oil. Sauté apples until tender but still firm. Add cider and simmer while cooking pork chops.

4. Heat 2 teaspoons olive oil in another large sauté pan. Add pork and sauté until browned on both sides. Spread champagne mustard on top of cutlets.

5. Sprinkle garlic and onions around chops. Add 1/2 cup white wine. Add beef broth and Worcestershire sauce. Stir to blend all ingredients around chops.

6. Cover and cook until onions are softened, about 5 minutes. Serve with sautéed apples on the side.

Calories 345
Calories from Fat 115
Total Fat 13.0 g
Saturated Fat 3.3 g
Trans Fat 0.0 g
Cholesterol 60 mg
Sodium 325 mg
Potassium 580 mg
Total Carbohydrate 34 g
Dietary Fiber 4 g
Sugars 25 g
Protein 22 g
Phosphorus 220 mg

Cook's Tips

QUICK–COOKING RICE CAN BE ADDED TO THE PORK CHOP PAN FOR A COMPLETE MEAL.

Pork Tenderloin with Mediterranean Crust

1 1/4–1 1/2 pounds pork tenderloin

1/4 cup stone-ground Dijon mustard

2 tablespoons dry marjoram

2 tablespoons dry basil leaves

4 cloves garlic, finely minced

1/2 teaspoon freshly ground pepper

This dish is quick and easy. It can be seasoned ahead of time and popped into the oven when guests arrive. The mustard herb coating allows for flavor in every bite without a sauce. Use a foil pan for no cleanup.

SERVES 4 | SERVING SIZE 1/4 recipe | EXCHANGES 4 Lean Meat

1. Preheat oven to 375°F.

2. Tuck narrow end of tenderloin under the thicker part and tie with butcher's twine for even cooking.

3. Coat pork with Dijon mustard.

4. Mix seasonings, garlic, and pepper. Coat pork tenderloin with seasoning mixture.

5. Roast in preheated oven until meat thermometer reaches 160°F, approximately 20 minutes. Let rest 10 minutes before slicing. Serve.

Calories 170
  Calories from Fat 35
Total Fat 4.0 g
  Saturated Fat 1.3 g
  Trans Fat 0.0 g
Cholesterol 75 mg
Sodium 415 mg
Potassium 515 mg
Total Carbohydrate 5 g
  Dietary Fiber 1 g
  Sugars 1 g
Protein 28 g
Phosphorus 270 mg

DAZZLING DINNER PARTIES

Radicchio & Romaine Ribbon Salad

1/2 head radicchio, cut into 1/4-inch thick ribbons

1 head romaine hearts cut into 1/4-inch-thick ribbons

1 fennel bulb, cut into julienned strips

1/4 cup Basic Vinaigrette (page 173) made with red wine vinegar

1/2 cup pomegranate seeds

I love this salad because it reminds me of Christmas ribbons that surround packages, with the pomegranate creating little jewels that would be in those packages, but it is good anytime of the year!

SERVES 4 | **SERVING SIZE** 1/4 recipe | **EXCHANGES** 1/2 Fruit, 1 Vegetable, 2 Fat

1. Place radicchio, romaine, fennel, and pomegranate in a large salad bowl. Add vinaigrette and toss well. Serve immediately.

Calories 130
  Calories from Fat 90
Total Fat 10.0 g
  Saturated Fat 1.3 g
  Trans Fat 0.0 g
Cholesterol 0 mg
Sodium 45 mg
Potassium 510 mg
Total Carbohydrate 11 g
  Dietary Fiber 4 g
  Sugars 5 g
Protein 2 g
Phosphorus 65 mg

Pecorino Romano Stuffed Meatballs

3 garlic cloves, minced

1 small onion, grated on box grater

2 large eggs

1 tablespoon chopped fresh basil

1/2 cup chopped fresh parsley

1 teaspoon Salt & Pepper Blend
(see page viii)

1 cup plain stuffing cubes

1/2 cup dry red wine

2 pounds extra lean (95%) ground
beef

2 ounces Pecorino Romano cheese,
cut into 20 small cubes

Placing a piece of Pecorino Romano in these meatballs makes them extra special for a dinner party. Pecorino is a very sharp sheep's milk cheese.

SERVES 20 | **SERVING SIZE** 1 meatball + 1/4 cup sauce
EXCHANGES 1/2 Carbohydrate, 2 Lean Meat

1. Preheat oven to 425°F; use convection if you have it.

2. Place all ingredients except the beef and Pecorino Romano in a large bowl. Mix well, add the beef, and gently mix. Roll into desired size meatballs. If the mixture does not hold together, add 1/4 cup additional stuffing cubes. Once you have the meatballs rolled, you can push a piece of the cheese inside each one and roll again to seal.

3. Place the meatballs on a parchment-lined baking sheet and bake in a very hot oven to brown the outside.

4. Place in Quick Marinara Sauce (see page 125) with an added 1/2 cup dry red wine. Simmer for at least 30 minutes or longer.

Cook's Tips

YOU DON'T WANT TO OVERMIX OR YOUR MEATBALLS WILL BE TOUGH. THIS IS WHY I LIKE TO MIX EVERYTHING BUT THE MEAT TOGETHER FIRST.

Calories 135
  Calories from Fat 55
Total Fat 6.0 g
  Saturated Fat 2.3 g
  Trans Fat 0.1 g
Cholesterol 50 mg
Sodium 450 mg
Potassium 485 mg
Total Carbohydrate 8 g
  Dietary Fiber 2 g
  Sugars 3 g
Protein 12 g
Phosphorus 150 mg

Roasted Beef Tenderloin

2 pounds lean beef tenderloin
1/4 teaspoon fine sea salt
1/4 teaspoon freshly ground pepper

This is one of the most elegant roasts you can serve to your guests and it really is simple to prepare. In fact, try not to cover up the great taste by overpowering it with strong spices. Sauces on the side complement it nicely.

SERVES 4 | SERVING SIZE 1/4 recipe | EXCHANGES 6 Lean Meat

1. Preheat oven to 400°F. You will need a roasting pan large enough to comfortably hold the meat.

2. Turn the skinny end under the roast and tie it so that the roast is an even circumference. Season with sea salt and freshly ground black pepper on all sides.

3. Place pork in roasting pan in the center of your oven and cook for approximately 30 minutes. After 30 minutes you will want to test for doneness. Rosy rare is 120–125°F. Medium is 140–145°F. This roast is best served rare or medium, but never well done. Serve with Rosemary Balsamic Onions (see page 172).

Cook's Tips

ASK THE BUTCHER TO TRIM ALL VISIBLE FAT.

RESTING TIME IS VERY IMPORTANT FOR ROASTING. WHEN THE ROAST IS DONE, LET IT REST AT LEAST 10–15 MINUTES, 25–30 IS BEST. IF SERVING IMMEDIATELY, SLICE AND PLATE. THIS IS A GOOD ITEM TO COOK EARLY IN THE DAY AND SERVE LATER AT ROOM TEMPERATURE. IF SERVING LATER, COOL ROAST COMPLETELY AND WRAP TIGHTLY IN FOIL. REFRIGERATE UNTIL 1 HOUR BEFORE SERVING TIME. UNWRAP, SLICE, AND PLATE.

Calories 280
  Calories from Fat 100
Total Fat 11.0 g
  Saturated Fat 4.4 g
  Trans Fat 0.0 g
Cholesterol 120 mg
Sodium 230 mg
Potassium 530 mg
Total Carbohydrate 0 g
  Dietary Fiber 0 g
  Sugars 0 g
Protein 42 g
Phosphorus 330 mg

DAZZLING DINNER PARTIES

Rosemary Garlic Chicken with Pasta

1 pound boneless, skinless chicken breasts

2 teaspoons no-salt garlic herb seasoning (I used McCormick)

4 cloves garlic, minced

1/4 cup fresh rosemary

1 cup chopped onion (about 1/2 of a large onion)

1 tablespoon extra virgin olive oil

1/2 pound whole-wheat farfalle pasta

4 cups chopped fresh plum tomatoes, about 9 or 10 tomatoes

2 cups pasta cooking water, reserved from cooking the pasta

4 ounces fresh arugula

This is a combination of a do-ahead and a one-dish meal. You can cook the pasta ahead, marinate the chicken, have all ingredients ready to go into the sauté pan, and then it becomes a one-dish meal.

SERVES 6 | SERVING SIZE 1/6 recipe | **EXCHANGES** 1 1/2 Starch, 2 Vegetable, 2 Lean Meat

1. Cut chicken into bite-sized pieces. Toss with garlic herb seasoning, garlic, rosemary, onion, and olive oil. Marinate about 30 minutes.

2. Cook pasta according to package directions, to al dente stage. When pasta is done, drain, reserving 2 cups of the pasta cooking water.

3. Place chicken mixture in large sauté pan. Heat and sauté until chicken is golden.

4. Add tomatoes and cook 3–5 minutes until tomatoes soften. Add pasta water and cook 10 minutes. Add pasta and cook another 3–5 minutes. Add the arugula just before serving and mix well.

Calories 275
Calories from Fat 45
Total Fat 5.0 g
Saturated Fat 1.0 g
Trans Fat 0.0 g
Cholesterol 45 mg
Sodium 60 mg
Potassium 590 mg
Total Carbohydrate 37 g
Dietary Fiber 5 g
Sugars 6 g
Protein 24 g
Phosphorus 260 mg

DAZZLING DINNER PARTIES

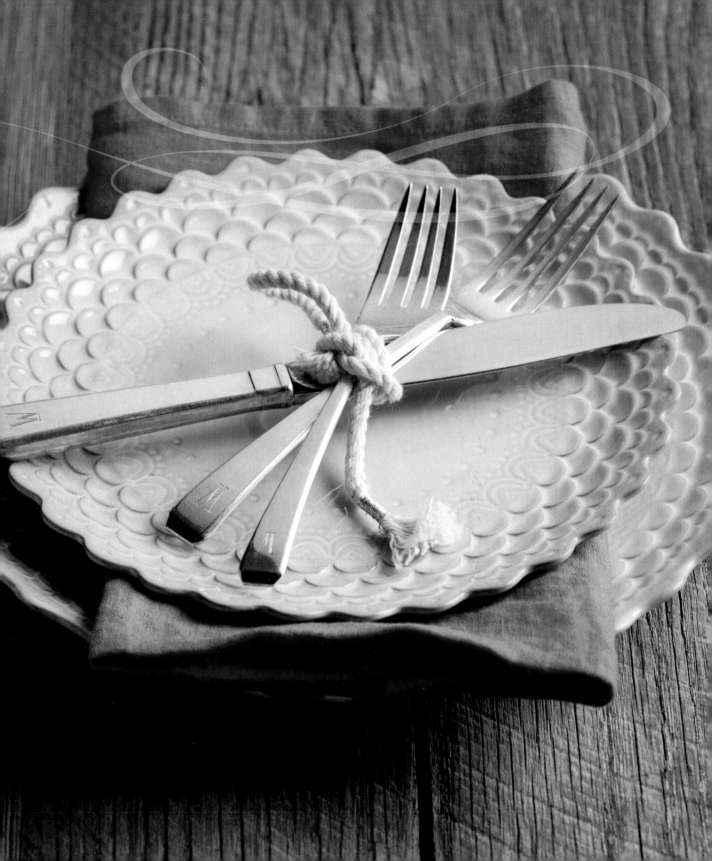

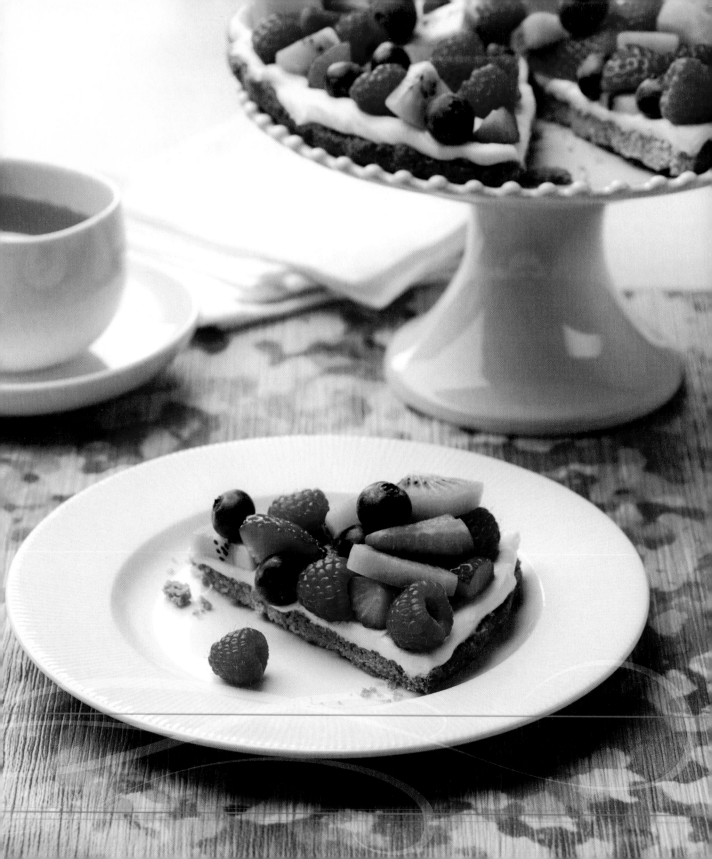

DESSERT PARTY

Baked Lemon Ricotta

1 lemon
3 large egg whites
1/2 teaspoon fine sea salt
1 pound light ricotta
Nonstick cooking spray

This dish is great served warm or cold and can be a "light" cheesecake for dessert. It could also double as an hors d'oeuvre.

SERVES 12 | SERVING SIZE 1/12 recipe | EXCHANGES 1 Lean Meat

1. Preheat oven to 350°F.
2. Zest lemon, cut it in half, and then juice it.
3. Separate eggs. Beat the egg whites until stiff peaks form.
4. Place the salt, lemon, eggs, and ricotta in a large bowl. Mix well. Transfer to a 6-inch round baking dish that has been sprayed with nonstick cooking spray or your own olive oil in a spray bottle.
5. Bake 30 minutes until the edges begin to brown.
6. Leave in the baking dish and add a small knife to the pan so that it can be sliced like a small cheesecake at the table.

Cook's Tips

CAN BE SERVED WARM OR COLD. THIS IS A DISH THAT CAN ALSO BE PART OF A DO-AHEAD MENU.

Calories 55
  Calories from Fat 20
Total Fat 2.5 g
  Saturated Fat 1.3 g
  Trans Fat 0.0 g
Cholesterol 55 mg
Sodium 175 mg
Potassium 70 mg
Total Carbohydrate 2 g
  Dietary Fiber 0 g
  Sugars 2 g
Protein 5 g
Phosphorus 95 mg

DESSERT PARTY

Blood Orange Olive Oil Cake

1 cup Splenda

1/2 cup extra virgin olive oil

1/2 cup blood orange Juice

1 egg, lightly beaten

2 egg whites, lightly beaten

2 cups all-purpose flour

1 tablespoon baking powder

1/2 teaspoon fine sea salt

Nonstick cooking spray

Confectioners sugar in a shaker or sifter

FOR CUPCAKES
Calories 175
  Calories from Fat 90
Total Fat 10.0 g
  Saturated Fat 1.4 g
  Trans Fat 0.0 g
Cholesterol 15 mg
Sodium 205 mg
Potassium 60 mg
Total Carbohydrate 19 g
  Dietary Fiber 1 g
  Sugars 3 g
Protein 3 g
Phosphorus 145 mg

FOR CAKE
Calories 135
  Calories from Fat 65
Total Fat 7.0 g
  Saturated Fat 1.1 g
  Trans Fat 0.0 g
Cholesterol 10 mg
Sodium 155 mg
Potassium 45 mg
Total Carbohydrate 14 g
  Dietary Fiber 0 g
  Sugars 2 g
Protein 3 g
Phosphorus 110 mg

Blood oranges are truly a treat, but if you cannot find them, you can use any citrus that you like. This cake makes a great presentation when baked in a shaped bundt pan.

CUPCAKES: SERVES 12 | **SERVING SIZE** 1 cupcake | **EXCHANGES** 1 1/2 Carbohydrate, 2 Fat
CAKE: SERVES 16 | **SERVING SIZE** 1/16 recipe | **EXCHANGES** 1 Carbohydrate, 1 1/2 Fat

1. Preheat oven to 350°F.

2. In a large bowl, cream Splenda, oil, and orange juice. Add the egg and egg whites and mix completely.

3. Combine flour, baking powder, and salt. Slowly add to above, until well blended.

4. Lightly spray cake pan with nonstick cooking spray. For cakelette or cupcakes, pour batter in pans to 3/4 full.

5. Bake 30 minutes for mini cakes or cupcakes or 50 minutes for cake, or until toothpick comes out clean. Cake pan sizes vary, so test carefully and adjust baking time accordingly.

6. Sprinkle with confectioners sugar and garnish with edible flowers or fruit.

Carrot Cake

2 1/4 cups all-purpose flour

2 teaspoons baking powder

1 1/2 teaspoons ground cinnamon

1/4 teaspoon salt

2 cups grated carrot

1/2 cup light (white) sugar blend (I used Domino light sugar and Stevia blend)

1/4 cup Splenda Brown Sugar Blend

1/4 cup canola oil

3 large eggs

1 teaspoon vanilla extract

1 cup plain, nonfat yogurt

Most people don't realize that carrot cake can be a fat- and sugar-laden dessert, but here we have a very low-fat, low-sugar version of an all-time favorite.

SERVES 16 | **SERVING SIZE** 1 slice | **EXCHANGES** 1 1/2 Carbohydrate, 1 Fat

1. Preheat oven to 350°F.

2. Combine flour, baking powder, cinnamon, and salt in medium bowl. Stir with whisk. Add carrot and mix well.

3. Place sugars and oil in large bowl. Beat with mixer at medium speed until well combined. Add eggs, 1 at a time, beating well. Add vanilla and beat into mixture. Add flour mixture and yogurt alternately. Spread batter into a bundt, tube, or angel food pan.

4. Bake 35–40 minutes until toothpick inserted comes out clean. For a finishing touch, you can sprinkle lightly with confectioners sugar once cake is completely cooled.

Calories 155
  Calories from Fat 40
Total Fat 4.5 g
  Saturated Fat 0.6 g
  Trans Fat 0.0 g
Cholesterol 35 mg
Sodium 115 mg
Potassium 115 mg
Total Carbohydrate 24 g
  Dietary Fiber 1 g
  Sugars 8 g
Protein 4 g
Phosphorus 125 mg

Nut-Crusted Fresh Fruit Tart

CRUST

1 cup old-fashioned rolled oats

1/4 cup all-purpose flour

1/4 cup ground walnuts

4 tablespoons trans-fat-free tub margarine (Smart Balance)

3 tablespoons honey

Water (as needed)

FILLING

8 ounces fat-free cream cheese

1/4 cup honey

TOPPING

2 pints fresh fruit (a mixture of berries is nice or any combination of your favorite fresh fruits)

This crunchy, fiber-filled crust needs to be made in time to cool before adding the filling and fruit, but don't worry, it only takes a few minutes.

SERVES 8 | **SERVING SIZE** 1 slice | **EXCHANGES** 2 1/2 Carbohydrate, 1 Fat

1. Preheat oven to 350°F.

2. Place oats, flour, and nuts in food processor. Pulse to mix. Add margarine and pulse until you have coarse crumbs. Add honey and pulse until mixture holds together. (If the mixture seems too stiff to press into a tart pan, add a few drops of water.)

3. Very gently, press the mixture into the bottom and up the sides of a 9-inch pie or tart pan. Bake 12–15 minutes, or until golden. Cool.

4. To prepare filling, mix cream cheese and honey together in food processor. Spread over cooled crust. Top with mounds of your favorite fresh fruit.

VARIATIONS:
- MIXED BERRIES
- CHOPPED MANGO AND SLICED KIWI
- CANNED PINEAPPLE AND MANDARIN ORANGES
- CAN ALSO BE MADE IN INDIVIDUAL TART PANS
- TRY GRATING SOME DARK CHOCOLATE OVER THE TOP BEFORE SERVING

Cook's Tips

BANANAS, APPLES, AND PEARS NEED TO BE DIPPED IN ACIDULATED WATER TO MAINTAIN FRESHNESS AND PREVENT BROWNING. ACIDULATED WATER IS WATER THAT HAS HAD A SQUEEZE OF FRESH LEMON OR LIME JUICE, OR A TABLESPOON OF VINEGAR ADDED TO IT.

SPRAY YOUR MEASURING CUP WITH NONSTICK COOKING SPRAY WHEN MEASURING HONEY OR PEANUT BUTTER.

Calories 225
  Calories from Fat 65
Total Fat 7.0 g
  Saturated Fat 1.5 g
  Trans Fat 0.0 g
Cholesterol 5 mg
Sodium 230 mg
Potassium 215 mg
Total Carbohydrate 36 g
  Dietary Fiber 4 g
  Sugars 21 g
Protein 6 g
Phosphorus 215 mg

DESSERT PARTY

Pumpkin Chiffon Ring

1 teaspoon ground cinnamon

3/4 teaspoon salt

1/2 teaspoon ground ginger

1/2 teaspoon ground nutmeg

1 1/4 cups cake flour

1 3/4 cups confectioners sugar, plus additional for dusting cake (divided use)

12–14 large egg whites to equal 1 2/3 cups

1 1/2 teaspoons cream of tartar

1 1/2 teaspoons vanilla extract

1 cup solid pack pumpkin (not pumpkin pie mix)

Nonstick cooking spray

This recipe was inspired by a fitness center recipe request. It has been a favorite of many of my friends for so long, I barely remember how it came to be!

SERVES 16 | **SERVING SIZE** 1 piece | **EXCHANGES** 1 1/2 Carbohydrate

1. Preheat oven to 375°F.

2. Mix cinnamon, salt, ginger, nutmeg, flour, and 3/4 cup confectioners sugar in a bowl, and set aside.

3. In large mixer bowl, beat egg whites and cream of tartar until soft peaks form. Add vanilla. Beating at high speed, sprinkle in 1 cup (2 tablespoons at a time) confectioners sugar, until sugar dissolves and whites stand in stiff peaks. Remove 1 cup egg whites to medium bowl and fold in pumpkin.

4. With rubber spatula or wire whisk, fold flour mixture into beaten egg whites in large bowl just until flour disappears. Then, gently fold in pumpkin mixture. Do not overmix.

5. Pour batter into 10–inch tube pan that has been sprayed with nonstick cooking spray. Bake 35 minutes or until cake springs back when lightly touched. Invert cake in pan on funnel or bottle and cool completely. This will keep cake from falling.

6. Loosen cake from pan. Place on serving plate and dust with additional confectioners sugar.

Calories 110
Calories from Fat 0
Total Fat 0.0 g
Saturated Fat 0.1 g
Trans Fat 0.0 g
Cholesterol 0 mg
Sodium 155 mg
Potassium 135 mg
Total Carbohydrate 23 g
Dietary Fiber 1 g
Sugars 14 g
Protein 4 g
Phosphorus 20 mg

DESSERT PARTY

Fresh Fruit & Ricotta Parfaits

1 1/2 cups reduced-fat ricotta cheese

2 tablespoons honey

2 teaspoons vanilla extract

4 cups fresh berries, such as a mixture of blueberries and raspberries

Fresh mint leaves (for garnish)

These parfaits are so pretty! For a festive breakfast, try adding a sprinkling of granola.

SERVES 6 | **SERVING SIZE** 1 parfait | **EXCHANGES** 1 1/2 Carbohydrate, 1/2 Fat

1. Mix cheese, honey, and vanilla.

2. Wash and dry berries.

3. Layer ricotta and berries in pretty serving dishes, such as stemmed wine glasses or a trifle dish. Garnish with fresh mint.

Calories 135
  Calories from Fat 30
Total Fat 3.5 g
  Saturated Fat 2.0 g
  Trans Fat 0.0 g
Cholesterol 20 mg
Sodium 150 mg
Potassium 185 mg
Total Carbohydrate 21 g
  Dietary Fiber 4 g
  Sugars 15 g
Protein 8 g
Phosphorus 130 mg

Typical Roman Cake

2 pounds fresh fat-free ricotta cheese

1 cup sugar blend for baking

1 cup flour

5 large eggs

2 teaspoons vanilla

3/4 cup dark chocolate chips

Nonstick cooking spray

This recipe is from a wonderful cooking class that I attended in the Trastevere section of Rome. The original recipe called for "a handful of flour" but I have found that 1 cup of flour gives the best results.

SERVES 16 | **SERVING SIZE** 1 slice
EXCHANGES 1/2 Fat-Free Milk, 1 1/2 Carbohydrate, 1/2 Fat

1. Mix all ingredients, except chocolate chips, with electric mixer until smooth. Add chocolate chips.

2. Pour mixture into a springform pan that has been sprayed with a nonstick cooking spray.

3. Bake at 375°F for 40 minutes or until top is golden brown.

Calories 185
Calories from Fat 35
Total Fat 4.0 g
Saturated Fat 2.0 g
Trans Fat 0.0 g
Cholesterol 80 mg
Sodium 70 mg
Potassium 135 mg
Total Carbohydrate 27 g
Dietary Fiber 0 g
Sugars 19 g
Protein 10 g
Phosphorus 155 mg

DESSERT
PARTY

Vanilla Yogurt Crumb Cake

1 cup Splenda

1/4 cup canola oil

1 egg, lightly beaten

2 egg whites, lightly beaten

1/2 cup nonfat cottage cheese

1/2 cup plain, nonfat yogurt

2 1/2 teaspoons vanilla extract

2 cups all-purpose flour, plus additional to lightly dust pan

1 tablespoon baking powder

Nonstick cooking spray

1/2 cup Crumb Topping (see page 163)

This old standby is made better for us with no-guilt yogurt and cottage cheese but still maintains a rich taste.

SERVES 12 | **SERVING SIZE** 1 slice | **EXCHANGES** 1 1/2 Carbohydrate, 1 1/2 Fat

1. Preheat oven to 350°F.

2. Cream Splenda and oil in mixer bowl. Add the egg and egg whites and mix completely.

3. Blend the cottage cheese in a blender and blend until smooth. Combine with yogurt. Pour into mixing bowl with sugar and oil mixture. Add vanilla.

4. Slowly add the flour and baking powder, stirring until blended.

5. Lightly spray a 10-inch tube pan and then dust with flour. Pour 2/3 of batter into pan. Sprinkle 1/2 Crumb Topping (page 163) over the batter. Pour in the remaining batter. Top with remaining crumb topping.

6. Bake 40–45 minutes or until toothpick inserted comes out clean.

⁓**VARIATIONS:** CAN BE MADE IN MUFFIN TINS; BAKE 15–20 MINUTES.

Calories 175
  Calories from Fat 65
Total Fat 7.0 g
  Saturated Fat 0.8 g
  Trans Fat 0.0 g
Cholesterol 15 mg
Sodium 160 mg
Potassium 85 mg
Total Carbohydrate 23 g
  Dietary Fiber 1 g
  Sugars 4 g
Protein 5 g
Phosphorus 190 mg

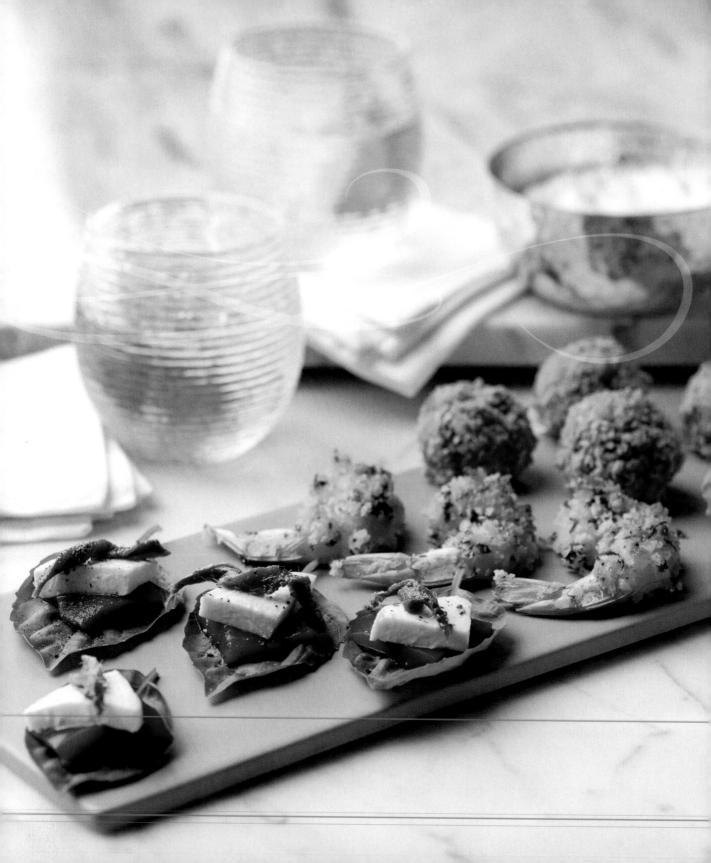

HORS D'OEUVRES

Apricot Walnut Bites

8 ounces goat cheese with fresh
   herbs

24 dried apricot halves

24 walnut halves

*These small bites are wonderful because there is so much
flavor packed into one little bite.*

SERVES 24 | **SERVING SIZE** 1/24 recipe | **EXCHANGES** 1 Fat

1. Slice goat cheese into 24 equal-size pieces. Place a piece of
   goat cheese on each apricot half and top with a walnut half.
   Refrigerate until serving time.

Calories 45
   Calories from Fat 30
Total Fat 3.5 g
   Saturated Fat 1.5 g
   Trans Fat 0.0 g
Cholesterol 10 mg
Sodium 45 mg
Potassium 50 mg
Total Carbohydrate 3 g
   Dietary Fiber 0 g
   Sugars 2 g
Protein 2 g
Phosphorus 35 mg

**HORS
D'OEUVRES**

Asiago & Speck Wine Crisps

2 ounces Speck Alto Adige IGP, chopped

2 ounces Asiago D'Allevo DOP, grated, equaling 1/2 cup

3 tablespoons unsalted butter, cut into thirds

1 teaspoon onion flakes

1 teaspoon Italian herb blend

1 cup unbleached flour

1 teaspoon baking powder

2 tablespoons extra virgin olive oil

2 egg whites (optional)

1/4 cup Asiago Pressato DOP

EQUIPMENT

Food processor

Parchment-lined baking sheets

Pastry brush

These crispy hors d'oeuvres are great with drinks or a glass of wine! Make them ahead and keep them in the freezer for unexpected company. You can freeze the baked crisps or the dough for fresh baked crisps without the prep.

SERVES 13 | SERVING SIZE 2 crisps | **EXCHANGES** 1/2 Starch, 1 Fat

1. Preheat oven to 375°F. Line baking sheets with parchment.

2. Place speck in food processor fitted with steel blade. Pulse a few times to make it very fine. Add cheese and butter and process until smooth.

3. Add flour and baking powder and pulse just until flour is blended in. This will look like coarse corn meal. Stream in extra virgin olive oil to bind, approximately 2–3 tablespoons.

4. Roll dough into balls and place on parchment–lined baking sheets. Brush with egg white and sprinkle with additional Asiago.

5. Bake 8–10 minutes until golden brown.

Calories 80
  Calories from Fat 35
Total Fat 4.0 g
  Saturated Fat 1.3 g
  Trans Fat 0.0 g
Cholesterol 5 mg
Sodium 155 mg
Potassium 45 mg
Total Carbohydrate 8 g
  Dietary Fiber 0 g
  Sugars 0 g
Protein 4 g
Phosphorus 80 mg

Cook's Tips

DOUGH CAN BE FROZEN OR CRISPS CAN BE BAKED AND FROZEN.

DO NOT LET PARCHMENT EXTEND BEYOND BAKING SHEET OR IT WILL BURN.

Asparagus Crêpes with Fresh Herb Cheese

FILLING

1 (8-ounce) package light Boursin cheese

1/4 cup fresh chives, chopped

1/4 cup flat Italian parsley, chopped

24 thin asparagus spears

BASIC CREPES
(to make 2 dozen, 4-inch crepes)

1 large egg

2 large egg whites

1 cup 2% milk

1/3 cup water

2 tablespoons extra virgin olive oil

1 cup unbleached, all-purpose flour

1/4 teaspoon fine sea salt

The crepe batter needs to rest for at least 30 minutes and up to 24 hours. Crepes can be made ahead and frozen or refrigerated.

SERVES 24 | SERVING SIZE 1 crepe with filling | EXCHANGES 1/2 Carbohydrate, 1/2 Fat

1. Bring Boursin cheese to room temperature. Mix Boursin cheese and herbs for filling. Set aside.

2. Whisk together eggs, egg whites, milk, water, and olive oil. Whisk in the flour and salt until all lumps have disappeared. Place in an airtight container. Refrigerate 30 minutes to 24 hours.

3. Wash asparagus and break off ends. Steam for 6 minutes. Remove from steamer and place in a bowl of ice–cold water to preserve color and prevent further cooking.

4. Heat pan to medium. Pour 2 tablespoons of batter in center and swirl around to make thin crepe. Cook until top is dry, approximately 1 minute. Using a rubber spatula, flip crepe and cook other side. Crepe will slide off pan when ready. Place on paper towel and repeat. Place paper towels between crepes.

5. Cut asparagus to appropriate length for crepes. Layer 1 crepe, 1/2–1 teaspoon cheese mixture, and 1 asparagus spear. Roll up and serve with additional fresh herb garnish.

Cook's Tips

CREPES CAN BE PREPARED UP TO 1 DAY AHEAD OR FROZEN FOR 2 WEEKS. WRAP TIGHTLY IN PLASTIC.

Calories 60
Calories from Fat 35
Total Fat 4.0 g
Saturated Fat 1.3 g
Trans Fat 0.0 g
Cholesterol 5 mg
Sodium 155 mg
Potassium 45 mg
Total Carbohydrate 8 g
Dietary Fiber 0 g
Sugars 0 g
Protein 4 g
Phosphorus 80 mg

HORS D'OEUVRES

Basil Cups with Roasted Red Pepper & Fresh Mozzarella

1 bunch fresh basil, washed and dried (large leaves are best)

1 pound fresh mozzarella, cut into 32, 1/4-inch-thick pieces

4 roasted red peppers, cut into 1-inch squares

Freshly ground pepper

4 tablespoons balsamic glaze

2 cans rolled anchovies with capers (optional)

Good-quality extra virgin olive oil (optional)

This appetizer/hors d'oeuvre is easy to prepare, colorful, and can be made early in the day.

SERVES 32 | **SERVING SIZE** 1/32 recipe | **EXCHANGES** 1 Lean Meat

1. Layer a basil leaf, a piece of mozzarella, and a piece of roasted red pepper. Sprinkle with freshly ground black pepper.

2. Cover and refrigerate until serving time. Just before serving, put a drop of balsamic glaze on each piece. Garnish with anchovies and olive oil, if desired.

Calories 45
Calories from Fat 20
Total Fat 2.5 g
Saturated Fat 1.5 g
Trans Fat 0.0 g
Cholesterol 5 mg
Sodium 75 mg
Potassium 60 mg
Total Carbohydrate 2 g
Dietary Fiber 0 g
Sugars 1 g
Protein 3 g
Phosphorus 60 mg

Bell Pepper Mélange

1 tablespoon extra virgin olive oil

1 small onion, thinly sliced, about 1/2 cup

2 bell peppers (about 8 ounces each), sliced as thinly as possible, and cut into 2-inch lengths

SERVES 8 | **SERVING SIZE** 1/4 cup | **EXCHANGES** 1 Vegetable

1. Place olive oil, onions, and peppers in a large sauté pan and cook until edges begin to brown, about 8–10 minutes.

2. Use as topping for Polenta Cheese Squares (page 110).

Calories 30
  Calories from Fat 20
Total Fat 2.0 g
  Saturated Fat 0.3 g
  Trans Fat 0.0 g
Cholesterol 0 mg
Sodium 0 mg
Potassium 110 mg
Total Carbohydrate 4 g
  Dietary Fiber 1 g
  Sugars 2 g
Protein 1 g
Phosphorus 15 mg

Crispy Frico

3 cups Parmigiano-Reggiano or Grana Padano cheese, coarsely grated

SERVES 48 | **SERVING SIZE** 1/48 recipe | **EXCHANGES** 1/2 Fat

1. Preheat oven 350°F. Line two sheet pans with a nonstick surface.

2. Place cheese onto pan liner, and spread out to a thin layer. Bake for 6–7 minutes or until golden.

3. Once Frico is cooked, let it cool for a few seconds. Carefully place it over a small inverted bowl until completely cooled.

Calories 20
  Calories from Fat 15
Total Fat 1.5 g
  Saturated Fat 1.1 g
  Trans Fat 0.0 g
Cholesterol 5 mg
Sodium 30 mg
Potassium 0 mg
Total Carbohydrate 0 g
  Dietary Fiber 0 g
  Sugars 0 g
Protein 2 g
Phosphorus 35 mg

HORS D'OEUVRES

Fresh Tomato & Basil Sauce

12 plum tomatoes

1/2 teaspoon fine sea salt

2 cloves garlic

1 tablespoon extra virgin olive oil

1/4 teaspoon freshly ground pepper

1 cup fresh basil leaves

This mixture makes a great topping for the Polenta Cheese Squares (page 110) or bruschetta, and there is no cooking required!

SERVES 8 | SERVING SIZE 1/8 recipe | EXCHANGES 1 Vegetable

1. Chop tomatoes into bite-sized pieces and place in medium bowl. Sprinkle with salt to bring out the flavor and juice. Let sit a few minutes. Meanwhile, finely mince the garlic. Add garlic, olive oil, and pepper to tomatoes. Tear basil leaves and add to tomato mixture.

2. Use as a topping for Polenta Cheese Squares (page 110). You can also toss with hot pasta.

Calories 35
Calories from Fat 20
Total Fat 2.0 g
Saturated Fat 0.3 g
Trans Fat 0.0 g
Cholesterol 0 mg
Sodium 155 mg
Potassium 250 mg
Total Carbohydrate 4 g
Dietary Fiber 1 g
Sugars 2 g
Protein 1 g
Phosphorus 25 mg

HORS D'OEUVRES

Garlicky Baked Shrimp

1 cup whole-wheat panko breadcrumbs

2 tablespoons finely chopped garlic

1/2 cup finely chopped flat leaf parsley

1/4 cup grated Parmigiano-Reggiano cheese

1/2 teaspoon fine sea salt

1/4 teaspoon freshly ground black pepper

2 tablespoons extra virgin olive oil

1 pound (about 20) large raw shrimp, peeled and deveined

3/4 cup dry white wine

SERVES 10 | **SERVING SIZE** 2 shrimp | **EXCHANGES** 1/2 Starch, 1 Lean Meat

1. Preheat oven to 350°F.

2. Mix panko, garlic, parsley, Parmigiano, salt, and pepper in pie plate. Add olive oil to bring together so breading will stick to shrimp. Breading should stick together a little but should not be moist.

3. Roll the shrimp one by one in the panko mixture and place in a 9 × 13–inch baking dish. Shrimp should be somewhat coated but not totally encrusted. Sprinkle any remaining breading over the shrimp in the pan.

4. Pour in enough white wine to cover the bottom of the pan. Bake for approximately 30 minutes.

Calories 95
  Calories from Fat 30
Total Fat 3.5 g
  Saturated Fat 0.9 g
  Trans Fat 0.0 g
Cholesterol 50 mg
Sodium 385 mg
Potassium 100 mg
Total Carbohydrate 6 g
  Dietary Fiber 1 g
  Sugars 0 g
Protein 8 g
Phosphorus 100 mg

HORS
D'OEUVRES

Goat Cheese Mousse with Pomegranate on Endive Spears

6 ounces goat cheese, such as Montrachet

3 ounces Neufchatel cheese (light cream cheese)

2 tablespoons fresh Italian parsley

1 tablespoon freshly grated orange zest

3-4 heads Belgian endive, washed and dried, leaves separated and kept whole

1 large pomegranate, seeded (you will only need about half of the seeds but you can save the rest to add to a green salad)

I love the burst of wonderful flavor that you get when you bite into a pomegranate seed. Pomegranates are packed with nutritional benefits, including antioxidants. If you want a shortcut to seeding the pomegranate, look for containers of pomegranate seeds (arils) in better grocery stores.

SERVES 36 | SERVING SIZE 1/36 recipe | EXCHANGES 1/2 Fat

1. Mix together goat cheese, cream cheese, parsley, and orange zest.

2. Place a teaspoon of goat cheese mousse on the wider end of the endive.

3. Top with 4–5 pomegranate seeds. Refrigerate until serving time.

Cook's Tips

A SPOON OR A PASTRY BAG WITH A LARGE STAR TIP CAN BE USED.

Calories 25
  Calories from Fat 15
Total Fat 1.5 g
  Saturated Fat 1.0 g
  Trans Fat 0.0 g
Cholesterol 5 mg
Sodium 30 mg
Potassium 40 mg
Total Carbohydrate 1 g
  Dietary Fiber 0 g
  Sugars 1 g
Protein 1 g
Phosphorus 20 mg

Lentil & Pomegranate Salsa

2 1/2 cups cooked lentils

1 cup chopped yellow tomato

1 cup pomegranate arils

1 cup chopped bell pepper, yellow, red, orange, or green

1/2 cup chopped fresh Italian parsley

1/2 teaspoon sea salt with herbs

1/2 teaspoon freshly ground black pepper

1/4 cup red wine vinegar

1/4 cup extra virgin olive oil

Serve this as a salsa with baked chips or as a condiment with any grilled protein. It is also excellent as an entrée for a light meal. For a shortcut you can also purchase "ready to eat" cooked lentils.

SERVES 20 | **SERVING SIZE** 1/4 cup | **EXCHANGES** 1/2 Carbohydrate, 1/2 Fat

1. Place all ingredients in a large bowl and mix well. The dressing will mix itself in the bowl.

Calories 65
Calories from Fat 25
Total Fat 3.0 g
Saturated Fat 0.4 g
Trans Fat 0.0 g
Cholesterol 0 mg
Sodium 25 mg
Potassium 155 mg
Total Carbohydrate 7 g
Dietary Fiber 3 g
Sugars 2 g
Protein 3 g
Phosphorus 50 mg

Shrimp Lettuce Wraps

1 pound cooked shrimp, chopped into bite-sized pieces

8 large lettuce leaves, Boston or bibb lettuce works well

8 teaspoons Asian peanut sauce

8 teaspoons julienne or matchstick carrots

8 teaspoons sliced scallions

Quick, simple, and delicious—you can assemble these ahead of time or put everything out for guests to prepare their own.

SERVES 8 | SERVING SIZE 1 wrap | **EXCHANGES** 2 Lean Meat

1. Place shrimp in bowl. Place all other ingredients in separate bowls.

2. Begin by laying a piece of lettuce on a plate. Top with shrimp, peanut sauce, carrots, and sprouts. Roll to enclose filling.

Cook's Tips

THIS ALSO WORKS WELL WITH LEFTOVER CHICKEN.

Calories 75
  Calories from Fat 10
Total Fat 1.0 g
  Saturated Fat 0.2 g
  Trans Fat 0.0 g
Cholesterol 105 mg
Sodium 170 mg
Potassium 225 mg
Total Carbohydrate 2 g
  Dietary Fiber 0 g
  Sugars 1 g
Protein 14 g
Phosphorus 155 mg

Mini Crab Cakes with Horseradish Sauce

CRAB CAKES

8 ounces pasteurized crabmeat, such as Phillips brand (backfin is best, lump is too large)

1/2 cup Italian-style breadcrumbs, plus additional 1/4 cup (if needed)

1/4 cup roughly chopped scallions or green onions

1 tablespoon fresh lemon juice

1/2 teaspoon hot sauce

1/4 teaspoon fine sea salt

2 egg whites

Few grinds fresh black pepper

1 cup cornflakes

DIPPING SAUCE

1/2 cup plain, low-fat yogurt

1 or 2 teaspoons prepared horseradish

SERVES 9 | SERVING SIZE 1 crab cake | **EXCHANGES** 1/2 Starch, 1 Lean Meat

1. Preheat oven to 450°F.

2. Mix all crab cake ingredients, except cornflakes, together. Mixture should be dry enough to form balls. If not, add more breadcrumbs.

3. Finely crush cornflakes in food processor.

4. Roll crab mixture into small balls and then into cornflakes. Bake on parchment–lined baking sheet until golden, approximately 10 minutes.

5. Drain yogurt through cheesecloth or coffee filter set in a colander for about 20 minutes. Mix with horseradish to taste. Serve crab cakes with horseradish sauce.

VARIATIONS:
- SERVE WITH COCKTAIL SAUCE.
- MAKE 3 LARGE CRAB CAKES TO SERVE AS AN ENTRÉE AND BAKE FOR 15–20 MINUTES, UNTIL GOLDEN

Calories 70
  Calories from Fat 10
Total Fat 1.0 g
  Saturated Fat 0.3 g
  Trans Fat 0.0 g
Cholesterol 35 mg
Sodium 285 mg
Potassium 155 mg
Total Carbohydrate 9 g
  Dietary Fiber 0 g
  Sugars 2 g
Protein 7 g
Phosphorus 90 mg

Cook's Tips

A SMALL ICE CREAM SCOOP MAKES PORTIONING EASIER AND ELIMINATES ROLLING EACH BALL INDIVIDUALLY.

Polenta Cheese Squares

3 cups water

1 1/2 cups polenta

1/2 teaspoon herb seasoned sea salt (I use Seasonello brand), or 1/2 teaspoon fine sea salt and a pinch of Italian herb blend

1/2 cup freshly grated Parmigiano-Reggiano cheese

This bite–sized cheesy polenta square is a great replacement for the bread or crackers usually used to hold great toppings, such as the Fresh Tomato & Basil Sauce (page 104), Caramelized Onions (page 164), the Zucchini and Tomato Mix (page 119), or the Bell Pepper Mélange (page 102).

SERVES 24 | **SERVING SIZE** 1 square | **EXCHANGES** 1/2 Starch

1. Bring water to a boil and whisk in polenta and salt. Cook and stir until thickened, about 5 minutes. Stir in cheese.

2. Spread polenta in a 9 × 13–inch sheet pan.

3. Cool. Cut into 24 squares. Top with one of the toppings above.

Calories 40
  Calories from Fat 5
Total Fat 0.5 g
  Saturated Fat 0.4 g
  Trans Fat 0.0 g
Cholesterol 0 mg
Sodium 35 mg
Potassium 15 mg
Total Carbohydrate 7 g
  Dietary Fiber 1 g
  Sugars 0 g
Protein 1 g
Phosphorus 20 mg

HORS D'OEUVRES

Prosciutto Rolls with Fresh Ricotta & Artichoke

4 ounces part-skim ricotta cheese (fresh if possible)

10 ounces frozen artichoke hearts, thawed and chopped

1/4 cup chopped Italian parsley

1/4 cup chopped black olives

1/4 cup chopped roasted red pepper

8 ounces sliced prosciutto (about 16 slices)

1/8 cup balsamic glaze or 1/4 cup balsamic vinegar reduced to a glaze (see Cook's Tip)

This idea came to me after a lovely party that my daughter-in-law gave. She created this delicious appetizer using slightly different ingredients. Here I have modified it to meet our needs.

SERVES 24 | **SERVING SIZE** 2 pieces | **EXCHANGES** 1 Lean Meat

1. Mix cheese, artichokes, parsley, olives, and roasted red pepper.

2. Lay a sheet of parchment paper on the work surface. Place 4 pieces of prosciutto on top to form a square. Spread 1/4 of the cheese mixture on top. Roll and wrap in parchment. Refrigerate for an hour or longer to make it easier to slice into pinwheels. Repeat this process a total of 4 times.

3. Slice each roll into 12 pieces. Place on platter and serve with a sprinkle of balsamic glaze.

Cook's Tips

YOU CAN PURCHASE A BALSAMIC GLAZE OR YOU CAN MAKE YOUR OWN BY REDUCING BALSAMIC VINEGAR. PLACE 1/4 CUP BALSAMIC VINEGAR IN A SMALL SAUCEPAN AND BRING TO A BOIL. BOIL FOR ABOUT 5–7 MINUTES, WATCHING CAREFULLY. YOU WILL KNOW IT'S DONE WHEN IT LIGHTLY COATS THE BACK OF A SPOON.

Calories 35
Calories from Fat 15
Total Fat 1.5 g
Saturated Fat 0.6 g
Trans Fat 0.0 g
Cholesterol 5 mg
Sodium 195 mg
Potassium 80 mg
Total Carbohydrate 2 g
Dietary Fiber 1 g
Sugars 1 g
Protein 4 g
Phosphorus 45 mg

HORS D'OEUVRES

111

Rosemary, Lemon & Garlic Baked Ricotta

2 tablespoons fresh rosemary, roughly chopped

1 clove garlic, finely minced

1/2 teaspoon fine sea salt

1/4 teaspoon freshly ground black pepper

3 large eggs whites

1 lemon, juiced

1 pound low-fat ricotta

Nonstick cooking spray

Light ricotta is a great staple in your fridge. When you are craving something "cheesy," this is a great substitute for higher-fat ingredients.

SERVES 12 | **SERVING SIZE** 1/12 recipe | **EXCHANGES** 1 Lean Meat

1. Preheat oven to 350°F.

2. Place rosemary, garlic, salt, and pepper on a cutting board and chop together. Take the side of your chef's knife and rub the ingredients onto the cutting board to make a paste.

3. Separate eggs and beat the egg whites until stiff peaks form.

4. Place the lemon, eggs whites, and ricotta in a large bowl. Add in the rosemary garlic mixture. Mix well. Transfer to a 6-inch baking dish that has been sprayed with nonstick cooking spray or your own olive oil in a spray bottle.

5. Bake 30 minutes until the edges begin to brown. Leave in the baking dish and add a small knife so that it can be sliced like a small cheesecake.

6. Can be served warm or cold. This is a dish that can also be part of a do-ahead menu.

Calories 55
Calories from Fat 20
Total Fat 2.5 g
Saturated Fat 1.3 g
Trans Fat 0.0 g
Cholesterol 55 mg
Sodium 175 mg
Potassium 70 mg
Total Carbohydrate 2 g
Dietary Fiber 0 g
Sugars 2 g
Protein 5 g
Phosphorus 95 mg

Savory Pecorino Cheese & Almond Hors D'oeuvre Cookies

1 large egg

2 egg whites

1/4 teaspoon fine sea salt

1 1/2 cups all-purpose flour

1 teaspoon freshly ground black pepper

1/2 cup freshly grated Pecorino cheese

1/2 cup finely chopped almonds

1 egg, beaten with a teaspoon of water for egg wash

I love having little treats like this in my home. When someone stops by, I can simply pull a few from my freezer and delight my guests with a warm treat.

SERVES 24 | **SERVING SIZE** 1 cookie | **EXCHANGES** 1/2 Starch, 1/2 Fat

1. Place all ingredients except almonds and last egg white in the food processor fitted with a steel blade. Mix until a ball forms.

2. Divide dough in half. Roll each half into a log about 2 inches thick. Freeze for about 20 minutes to make it easier to slice. Roll each log into half of the almonds. Slice into 1/4–inch–thick slices. Place on parchment–lined baking sheets. Brush with the egg wash.

3. Bake at 375°F for 10 minutes.

Cook's Tips

CAN BE BAKED AND FROZEN OR FROZEN BEFORE BAKING.

Calories 55
  Calories from Fat 20
Total Fat 2.0 g
  Saturated Fat 0.6 g
  Trans Fat 0.0 g
Cholesterol 15 mg
Sodium 70 mg
Potassium 35 mg
Total Carbohydrate 7 g
  Dietary Fiber 0 g
  Sugars 0 g
Protein 2 g
Phosphorus 40 mg

Shrimp in Mustard Sauce

2 pounds medium shrimp, peeled and deveined

2 teaspoons salt

1/4 cup finely chopped Italian parsley

2 tablespoons capers

1/4 cup finely chopped shallots

1 clove garlic, peeled and crushed

1/4 cup tarragon vinegar (available in most supermarkets)

1/4 cup red wine vinegar

1/2 cup olive oil

4 tablespoons Dijon mustard

2 teaspoons crushed red pepper (Don't worry, it will not be too spicy)

I owe this recipe to my dear friends, Val and Laurie. They prepare it regularly for guests and it is always a hit. If you need a shortcut, you can purchase the shrimp already cooked, but don't tell Val and Laurie!

SERVES 16 | **SERVING SIZE** 1/16 recipe | **EXCHANGES** 1 Lean Meat, 1 1/2 Fat

1. Bring a large pot of water to a boil. Add 2 teaspoons salt to water and then shrimp. Boil until shrimp are pink, about 3 to 5 minutes, do not overcook. Drain and set aside.

2. Mix remaining ingredients in a large bowl. Add the cooked shrimp. Mix well. Refrigerate several hours or overnight.

Calories 105
  Calories from Fat 65
Total Fat 7.0 g
  Saturated Fat 1.1 g
  Trans Fat 0.0 g
Cholesterol 70 mg
Sodium 425 mg
Potassium 80 mg
Total Carbohydrate 2 g
  Dietary Fiber 0 g
  Sugars 0 g
Protein 8 g
Phosphorus 105 mg

HORS D'OEUVRES

Sophia & Barb's Mushroom-Filled Phyllo Triangles

3 (14 × 18-inch) phyllo sheets

10 ounces cremini mushrooms

1 large shallot

2 small cloves garlic

1/2 teaspoon fine sea salt

Few grinds of black pepper

1/4 cup fresh herbs, such as thyme and basil

1 tablespoon extra virgin olive oil

4 ounces light cream cheese (Neufchatel)

Nonstick cooking spray or your olive oil mister

This is a wonderful hors d'oeuvre to have in your freezer. All the work is done ahead of time and it's a special treat for both the guests and the host or hostess. My daughter-in-law and I developed this recipe together, which made it a very special treat for me.

SERVES 12 | SERVING SIZE 1 triangle | EXCHANGES 1/2 Carbohydrate, 1/2 Fat

1. Defrost phyllo in refrigerator for at least 3 hours. Do not defrost in microwave, as it will become gummy.

2. Wipe mushrooms with damp paper towel to remove any debris. Cut a fine sliver off the end of the stem and quarter the mushrooms.

3. Peel and quarter the shallot. Crush and peel garlic.

4. Fit food processor with steel blade. Place mushrooms, shallot, and garlic in food processor. Pulse to a finely chopped mixture. Add salt, pepper, and herbs and pulse once more.

5. Place olive oil in a large sauté pan and cook mushroom mixture until soft, approximately 5 minutes. Turn pan off and add cream cheese and mix well.

6. Unwrap defrosted phyllo and lay on parchment-lined work surface, such as your kitchen counter. Cover with plastic wrap and a damp towel to prevent phyllo from drying out.

7. Take 1 leaf of phyllo and place it on a parchment-lined surface. Spray with mister and add another leaf. Repeat for 3 leaves. Cut into 2-inch strips. Place 1 tablespoon of mushroom mixture on bottom end of phyllo and fold a triangle shape over the rest of the phyllo. Repeat until you have wrapped the length of phyllo and made a triangle. (It is like folding a flag.)

8. Place triangles on a parchment-lined baking sheet. Bake the phyllo at 375°F for 8–10 minutes.

Calories 60
  Calories from Fat 30
Total Fat 3.5 g
  Saturated Fat 1.4 g
  Trans Fat 0.0 g
Cholesterol 5 mg
Sodium 165 mg
Potassium 135 mg
Total Carbohydrate 6 g
  Dietary Fiber 0 g
  Sugars 1 g
Protein 2 g
Phosphorus 50 mg

HORS D'OEUVRES

115

Spinach & Artichoke Dip

5 ounces chopped frozen spinach (one half of a box)

14 ounces frozen artichokes

1 cup part-skim ricotta cheese

1 cup shredded part-skim mozzarella cheese

1/4 cup grated Parmigiano-Reggiano cheese

This classic party dip is even more delicious when prepared with ricotta instead of the higher-fat cream cheese and sour cream. If you have a small hors d'œuvre crockpot, bake the mixture in the removable crock and keep it warm by placing the removable crock back into the warming unit.

SERVES 28 | SERVING SIZE 2 tablespoons | EXCHANGES 1/2 Fat

1. Defrost spinach and squeeze out excess water. Defrost artichokes and chop.

2. Place all ingredients in a medium mixing bowl and mix thoroughly. Transfer to baking dish. Bake at 375°F for 20–30 minutes or until golden and bubbly.

Calories 30
  Calories from Fat 15
Total Fat 1.5 g
  Saturated Fat 1.0 g
  Trans Fat 0.0 g
Cholesterol 5 mg
Sodium 50 mg
Potassium 70 mg
Total Carbohydrate 2 g
  Dietary Fiber 1 g
  Sugars 0 g
Protein 3 g
Phosphorus 50 mg

HORS D'OEUVRES

Stuffed Mushrooms

10-ounce package of cremini mushrooms

1 tablespoon extra virgin olive oil

1 medium onion, minced

2 cloves garlic, minced

2 cups baby spinach, roughly chopped

1 cup plain breadcrumbs

1 1/2 cups low-sodium vegetable stock (divided use)

1 cup Parmigiano-Reggiano cheese, finely grated (divided use)

These delicious, savory mushrooms are an elegant hors d'oeuvre. I also like to serve them on a bed of sautéed spinach with olive oil and garlic for pizazz.

SERVES 15 | **SERVING SIZE** 1 mushroom | **EXCHANGES** 1/2 Carbohydrate, 1/2 Fat

1. Wipe mushrooms with damp paper towel. Trim bottom of stem and separate stems from mushrooms. Chop stems. Set mushroom caps aside.

2. Place olive oil in a large nonstick skillet. Add minced onion and garlic. Cook until onion becomes translucent.

3. Add mushroom stems and baby spinach. Cook 3 minutes to soften mushroom stems.

4. Add breadcrumbs and 1 cup stock. Heat thoroughly. Remove from heat. Add 1/2 cup Parmigiano–Reggiano and blend well.

5. Fill mushroom caps with mixture and place in baking dish. Add approximately 1/2 cup additional stock to baking dish. Cover with foil and bake in 350°F oven for 20–30 minutes until mushroom caps are tender.

6. Sprinkle with additional 1/2 cup Parmigiano–Reggiano cheese.

Cook's Tips

SERVE ON SAUTÉED BABY SPINACH AND DRIZZLE WITH BALSAMIC GLAZE.

Calories 70
Calories from Fat 25
Total Fat 3.0 g
Saturated Fat 1.4 g
Trans Fat 0.0 g
Cholesterol 5 mg
Sodium 110 mg
Potassium 175 mg
Total Carbohydrate 8 g
Dietary Fiber 1 g
Sugars 1 g
Protein 3 g
Phosphorus 85 mg

Stuffed Mushrooms with Pancetta

10-ounce package of cremini mushrooms

1 tablespoon extra virgin olive oil

4 ounces chopped pancetta

1 medium onion, minced

2 cloves garlic, minced

2 cups baby spinach, roughly chopped

1 cup plain breadcrumbs

1 1/2 cups low-sodium vegetable stock (divided use)

1/3 cup Parmigiano-Reggiano cheese, finely grated

SERVES 15 | SERVING SIZE 1 stuffed mushroom | EXCHANGES 1/2 Carbohydrate, 1 Fat

1. Clean mushrooms. Trim bottom of stem and separate stems from mushrooms. Chop stems. Set mushroom caps aside.

2. Place olive oil in a large nonstick skillet. Heat and add chopped pancetta, minced onion, and garlic. Cook until onion becomes translucent.

3. Add mushroom stems and baby spinach. Cook 3 minutes to soften mushroom stems.

4. Add breadcrumbs and 1 cup stock. Heat thoroughly.

5. Fill mushroom caps with mixture and place in baking dish. Add approximately 1/2 cup additional stock to baking dish. Cover with foil and bake in 350°F oven for 20–30 minutes until mushroom caps are tender. Sprinkle with Parmigiano–Reggiano cheese.

Calories 80
Calories from Fat 35
Total Fat 4.0 g
Saturated Fat 1.4 g
Trans Fat 0.0 g
Cholesterol 10 mg
Sodium 225 mg
Potassium 210 mg
Total Carbohydrate 8 g
Dietary Fiber 1 g
Sugars 1 g
Protein 4 g
Phosphorus 95 g

Zucchini & Tomato Mix

1 tablespoon extra virgin olive oil

2 cloves garlic, finely minced

1 medium zucchini, sliced (about 2 cups)

4 plum tomatoes, diced

1/2 teaspoon fine sea salt

1/4 teaspoon freshly ground pepper

1 cup fresh basil leaves

This mixture makes a great topping for the Polenta Cheese Squares (page 110) or bruschetta.

SERVES 8 | **SERVING SIZE** 1/3 cup | **EXCHANGES** 1 Vegetable

1. Place olive oil in large sauté pan. Add garlic and zucchini and cook until zucchini slices begins to wilt. Add tomatoes. Remove pan from heat. Stir in salt, pepper, and fresh basil. Cool.

Calories 30
  Calories from Fat 20
Total Fat 2.0 g
  Saturated Fat 0.3 g
  Trans Fat 0.0 g
Cholesterol 0 mg
Sodium 150 mg
Potassium 175 mg
Total Carbohydrate 3 g
  Dietary Fiber 1 g
  Sugars 1 g
Protein 1 g
Phosphorus 25 mg

HORS
D'OEUVRES

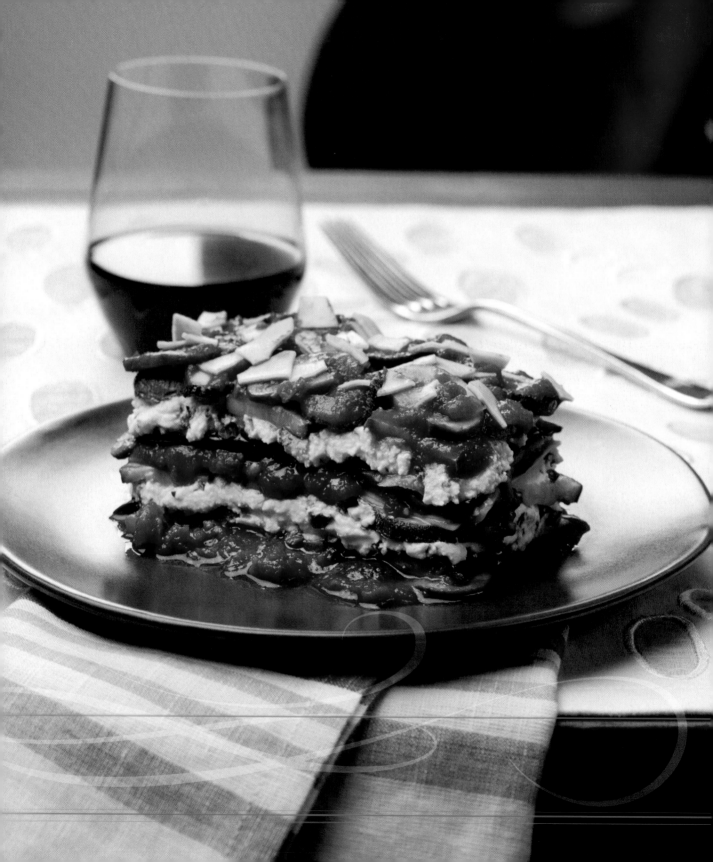

ITALIAN NIGHT

Individual Eggplant Parmigiano

MARINARA SAUCE

2 tablespoons extra virgin olive oil

2 cloves garlic, chopped

2 (28-ounce) cans no-salt-added tomato puree or crushed tomatoes

1 cup fresh basil leaves

EGGPLANT

1 eggplant (about 1 1/4 pounds)

3 large eggs

1 cup Italian-style breadcrumbs

1/4 cup grated Parmesan cheese

1 1/2 teaspoons Salt & Pepper Blend (page viii)

1/4 cup shredded part-skim mozzarella cheese (optional)

SERVES 12 | SERVING SIZE 1 slice eggplant + 1/2 cup marinara sauce
EXCHANGES 1/2 Starch, 3 Vegetable, 1 Fat

1. Preheat oven to 400°F.

2. Place a little olive oil in the bottom of a large saucepan, enough to cover the bottom. Add garlic and cook until fragrant, but not dark brown. Add tomatoes and basil. Bring to a low boil, then turn to simmer to cook.

3. Slice eggplant 1/2-inch thick. Lightly salt. This will prevent eggplant from absorbing too much olive oil.

4. Scramble eggs in large dish or pie plate.

5. Place breadcrumbs, Parmesan cheese, and Salt & Pepper Blend in large dish or pie plate. Mix well.

6. Dip eggplant in egg and then breadcrumbs. Place on parchment-lined baking sheet. Bake about 20 minutes or until eggplant is golden brown.

7. Top with about 1/2 cup marinara sauce and mozzarella cheese, if desired. Return to oven to melt cheese.

Calories 155
  Calories from Fat 45
Total Fat 5.0 g
  Saturated Fat 1.4 g
  Trans Fat 0.0 g
Cholesterol 50 mg
Sodium 430 mg
Potassium 700 mg
Total Carbohydrate 23 g
  Dietary Fiber 4 g
  Sugars 8 g
Protein 7 g
Phosphorus 120 mg

ITALIAN NIGHT

Beef Bracciole

8 pieces beef top round (about 2 pounds)

1/4 teaspoon fine sea salt

1/2 teaspoon freshly ground black pepper

1/2 teaspoon garlic powder

1/3 cup grated Grana Padano

2 cups fresh arugula

1 tablespoon extra virgin olive oil

4 cups Quick Marinara Sauce (see page 125)

1/2 cup dry red wine (preferably Italian wine)

Italian families will usually have their own favorite way to prepare this dish. I am giving you a very simple version that can be varied by changing the arugula to a preferred herb or spinach and using the cheese of your choosing.

SERVES 8 | SERVING SIZE 1/8 recipe | EXCHANGES 2 Vegetable, 3 Lean Meat, 1 Fat

1. Lay beef out on a large cutting board or piece of parchment paper. Lightly pound the meat with a flat meat pounder. This will help make it more tender.

2. Sprinkle with salt, pepper, and garlic powder. Using your fingers, distribute evenly over beef. Sprinkle Grana Padano and arugula evenly over beef.

3. Roll beef and secure each roll with a toothpick or two.

4. Place extra virgin olive oil in sauté pan large enough to hold all bracciole. Heat and add bracciole. Brown on all sides, about 5–10 minutes. Add marinara sauce and wine and simmer at least 1 hour (the longer, the better).

Calories 240
  Calories from Fat 90
Total Fat 10.0 g
  Saturated Fat 2.7 g
  Trans Fat 0.0 g
Cholesterol 60 mg
Sodium 585 mg
Potassium 765 mg
Total Carbohydrate 10 g
  Dietary Fiber 3 g
  Sugars 5 g
Protein 27 g
Phosphorus 235 mg

Bolognese-Style Pasta Sauce

2 tablespoons extra virgin olive oil

2 pounds ground bison

1 medium onion, chopped (about 3/4 cup)

3 cloves garlic, chopped

1/2 cup grated carrot

1/2 cup finely chopped celery

1/2 cup fresh basil, chopped

1/2 cup chopped Italian parsley

1 cup dry red wine, preferably Italian, such as Sangiovese or a red table wine

4 cups fresh plum tomatoes or 28 ounces canned, crushed tomatoes

I like to make this Bolognese-style sauce with American buffalo, also known as bison, because it has no saturated fat. It is also delicious with ground turkey breast or extra-lean ground beef.

SERVES 8 | SERVING SIZE 1 cup sauce | **EXCHANGES** 1 Vegetable, 3 Lean Meat, 1/2 Fat

1. Place extra virgin olive oil in large saucepan. Break up the bison and add to the pan in a single layer. Brown the bison. Do this in batches if you don't have a pan large enough to hold the meat in a thin layer.

2. Add onion, garlic, carrots, celery, and herbs. Cook 3 minutes and then add the red wine to deglaze the pan. Add the tomatoes and simmer 60–90 minutes.

Calories 185
  Calories from Fat 55
Total Fat 6.0 g
  Saturated Fat 1.3 g
  Trans Fat 0.0 g
Cholesterol 70 mg
Sodium 65 mg
Potassium 620 mg
Total Carbohydrate 7 g
  Dietary Fiber 2 g
  Sugars 4 g
Protein 26 g
Phosphorus 215 mg

ITALIAN NIGHT

Quick Marinara Sauce

1 tablespoon extra virgin olive oil

4 cloves garlic, minced

1/2 cup chopped fresh basil

1/2 cup chopped marjoram or oregano

28 ounces diced canned tomatoes or 12 fresh plum tomatoes, chopped

1/4 teaspoon fine sea salt

1/2 teaspoon freshly ground pepper

Additional basil, as desired

SERVES 4 | SERVING SIZE 1/2 cup | EXCHANGES 2 Vegetable, 1/2 Fat

1. Place olive oil in 4–6–quart saucepan. Add garlic and cook until fragrant. When garlic begins to turn brown, add basil, marjoram, tomatoes, salt, and pepper. Simmer 20 minutes. Add more basil if desired. Simmer 10 minutes more or longer.

Cook's Tips

THIS IS SUITABLE FOR ANY RECIPE CALLING FOR MARINARA. IT MAKES A GREAT PIZZA SAUCE OR PASTA SAUCE AND IS WONDERFUL WITH MEATBALLS.

Calories 75
  Calories from Fat 35
Total Fat 4.0 g
  Saturated Fat 0.5 g
  Trans Fat 0.0 g
Cholesterol 0 mg
Sodium 430 mg
Potassium 445 mg
Total Carbohydrate 10 g
  Dietary Fiber 3 g
  Sugars 5 g
Protein 2 g
Phosphorus 50 mg

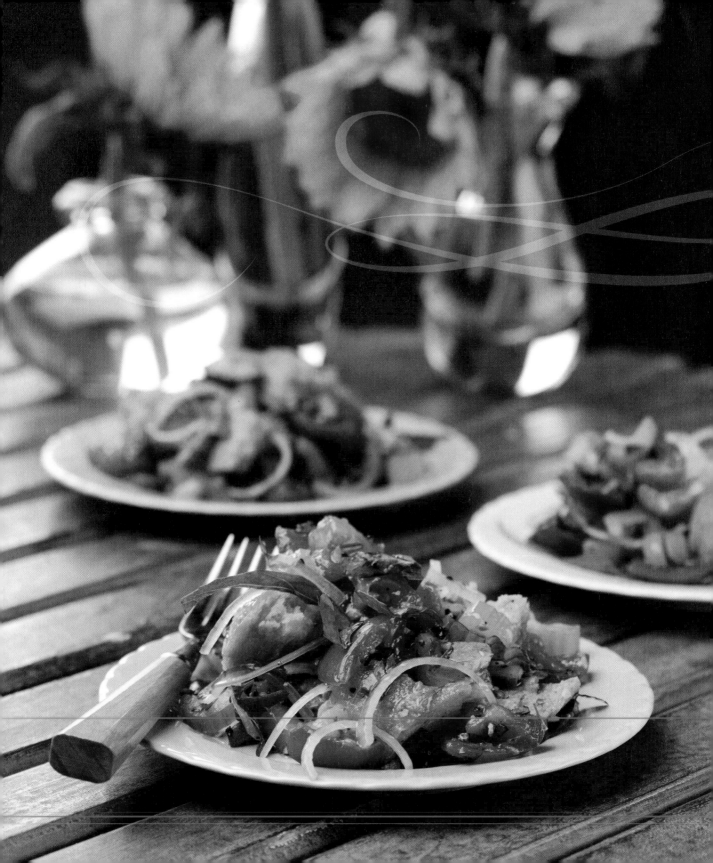

Classic Italian Panzanella (Bread & Tomato Salad)

2 medium tomatoes, cut into 1-inch cubes, or equivalent cherry tomatoes, cut in half

1/2 teaspoon fine sea salt

2 cups stale pieces of good quality Italian bread (such as a multigrain ciabatta)

1 cup cucumber, quartered lengthwise and thinly sliced (about 1/2 of an English cucumber)

2 stalks celery, sliced 1/2 inch thick

1 small red onion, cut in half and thinly sliced

1/4 teaspoon freshly ground black pepper

2 tablespoons red wine vinegar

2 tablespoons extra virgin olive oil

1/2 cup fresh basil leaves, torn into strips

1 cup flat Italian parley leaves, roughly chopped

This is a classic Italian salad that I had during my travels throughout Italy. Each cook puts their own special touch on the dish, but the main ingredients, like tomatoes, bread, celery, and onion, stay the same. If you often end up with leftover artisan bread, freeze it and save it for this salad.

SERVES 4 | **SERVING SIZE** 1/4 recipe | **EXCHANGES** 1 Starch, 1 Vegetable, 1 1/2 Fat

1. Place tomatoes in large salad bowl and sprinkle with salt. Let stand 5 minutes.

2. Break up bread and add to tomatoes. Add remaining salad ingredients and mix well.

Calories 165
  Calories from Fat 70
Total Fat 8.0 g
  Saturated Fat 1.2 g
  Trans Fat 0.0 g
Cholesterol 0 mg
Sodium 455 mg
Potassium 455 mg
Total Carbohydrate 21 g
  Dietary Fiber 3 g
  Sugars 5 g
Protein 4 g
Phosphorus 80 mg

Country Pork with Chickpeas

2 tablespoons extra virgin olive oil

2 pounds boneless, country spare ribs or pork loin cut into serving-size pieces

1 teaspoon Italian sea salt with herbs

1/2 teaspoon freshly ground black pepper

1 large onion, roughly chopped

4 garlic cloves, crushed

1 (15-ounce) can low-sodium chicken broth

1–2 cups Quick Marinara Sauce (see page 125)

1 (15-ounce) can low-sodium chickpeas, drained and rinsed

This is a perfect do-ahead dish. It is even more delicious when prepared a day or two ahead. Once the initial cooking is done and you get to the simmering stage, you can transfer to a crockpot and cook on high for 4 hours or low for 8 hours.

A Tre Colore Salad (see page 64) or asparagus with vinaigrette would complete the meal.

SERVES 7 | SERVING SIZE 1/7 recipe
EXCHANGES 1/2 Starch, 1 Vegetable, 4 Lean Meat, 1 1/2 Fat

1. Heat oil in large skillet or chef's pan. Add pork and season with salt and pepper. Brown on first side. Turn to cook second side and add onion and garlic to pan surface. Cook until pork and onions are golden brown.

2. Add stock to deglaze pan. Stir to loosen browned bits. Add marinara sauce and chickpeas. Mix well. Cook a minimum of 60 minutes or longer until pork is tender.

3. Serve over polenta made according to package directions.

Cook's Tips

WHEN I HAVE LEFTOVER CHEESES THAT I THINK MIGHT NOT KEEP WELL, I PLACE THEM IN MY FOOD PROCESSOR AND SHRED THEM AND THEN FREEZE THEM FOR DISHES LIKE THIS ONE.

Calories 305
  Calories from Fat 125
Total Fat 14.0 g
  Saturated Fat 3.7 g
  Trans Fat 0.0 g
Cholesterol 70 mg
Sodium 340 mg
Potassium 665 mg
Total Carbohydrate 16 g
  Dietary Fiber 4 g
  Sugars 5 g
Protein 28 g
Phosphorus 270 mg

ITALIAN NIGHT

Eggplant & Zucchini Lasagna

SAUCE

1 tablespoon extra virgin olive oil

2 cloves garlic, minced

1 teaspoon Italian seasoning blend

10 ounces cremini mushrooms, thinly sliced

28 ounces crushed tomatoes

1 teaspoon fine sea salt

1/2 teaspoon freshly ground black pepper

EGGPLANT & ZUCCHINI

1/2 teaspoon fine sea salt

1 1/4 pound eggplant, unpeeled, sliced into approximately 12 slices

1 pound (2 medium) zucchini, sliced into rounds

Olive oil cooking spray

FILLING & PASTA

1 pound fat-free ricotta

1 large egg

1 cup shredded part-skim mozzarella

1/4 cup grated Parmigiano-Reggiano cheese

1/4 teaspoon fine sea salt

1/2 cup chopped flat Italian Parsley

1/2 pound box no-boil lasagna noodles

Calories 195
  Calories from Fat 40
Total Fat 4.5 g
  Saturated Fat 1.7 g
  Trans Fat 0.0 g
Cholesterol 35 mg
Sodium 545 mg
Potassium 545 mg
Total Carbohydrate 27 g
  Dietary Fiber 4 g
  Sugars 8 g
Protein 13 g
Phosphorus 230 mg

In this recipe, I've replaced some of the pasta with sliced zucchini and eggplant so we get our veggies while still enjoying a great lasagna. Prepare the sauce first and then let it simmer while you are preparing the remaining parts of the dish.

SERVES 12 | SERVING SIZE 1 3 × 3 1/4-inch piece
EXCHANGES 1 Starch, 2 Vegetable, 1 Lean Meat, 1/2 Fat

1. Place olive oil in large saucepan. Add garlic, seasoning blend, and mushrooms and cook until garlic is fragrant and mushrooms begin to soften. Add tomatoes. Rinse the can with a little water and add to the pot. Add salt and pepper. Bring to a boil and then reduce heat to low. Simmer while preparing the lasagna.

2. Preheat broiler. Rub salt into eggplant slices. Let sit 10 minutes. Place eggplant and zucchini in single layer on parchment-lined baking sheet. Spray with cooking spray. Broil 5 minutes until they begin to brown.

3. Mix all filling ingredients except lasagna noodles in large bowl.

4. Place 1/3 of the sauce in a 9 x 13–inch baking dish. Place 3 lasagna noodles in pan. Layer a single layer of eggplant and zucchini over the noodles. Layer 1/2 of the cheese filling. Repeat. Break the last noodle into bite–sized pieces and sprinkle over the top. Top with remaining 1/3 sauce.

5. Place in preheated 350°F oven. Bake 20–30 minutes until bubbly. Cool at least 10 minutes before serving for neater slices.

Nonna's Baked Artichokes

1 cup whole-wheat panko breadcrumbs (plain unseasoned breadcrumbs can be substituted, but the texture of the dish will be far less crunchy)

2 tablespoons finely chopped garlic

1/2 cup finely chopped Italian flat leaf parsley

1/4 cup grated Parmigiano-Reggiano cheese

1/2 teaspoon fine sea salt

1/2 teaspoon freshly ground black pepper

1/4 cup extra virgin olive oil

4 pounds baby artichokes (about 2 packages)

1/2 lemon squeezed into large bowl of water (acidulated water to preserve color)

1/2 cup chicken or vegetable stock

My cooking buddy Val and I often share recipes. My favorites are those that he gives me from his mother, who was from Puglia, Italy.

SERVES 10 | **SERVING SIZE** 1/10 recipe | **EXCHANGES** 1/2 Starch, 1 Vegetable, 1 Fat

1. Preheat oven to 375°F.

2. Place panko, garlic, parsley, Parmigiano, salt, and pepper in a bowl. Add the 1/4 cup of olive oil and mix well. The mixture should come together in a loose paste–not enough to form a ball, but enough to slightly stick together when squeezed lightly.

3. Trim artichokes of all tough fibrous leaves, leaving only the white tender leaves. Trim stems of whatever fibrous outer skin there may be. If desired, stems may be discarded, but if trimmed well, they are very good. Cut baby artichokes in half and drop into acidulated water to prevent browning during remaining prep. If using mature artichokes, after removing choke, slice them lengthwise into approximate 1/4–inch slices and drop into acidulated solution until ready to cook. Once artichokes are trimmed, drain in a colander and then arrange in a 9 × 13–inch glass baking dish so that they sit in one layer, just slightly overlapping. Cover artichokes with the breadcrumb mixture. Pour about 1/4 inch of chicken stock or water into the dish.

4. Place uncovered dish in the oven and bake until the thickest part of the artichoke is slightly fork tender. Baking times will vary according to the artichoke used but 25–30 minutes should be the minimum, while mature artichokes may take up to 45 minutes. Personal taste will dictate the degree of doneness.

5. Remove from oven and allow to rest for at least 10 minutes. Can be served warm, at room temperature, or slightly cold from the fridge.

Calories 125
Calories from Fat 55
Total Fat 6.0 g
Saturated Fat 1.2 g
Trans Fat 0.0 g
Cholesterol 0 mg
Sodium 190 mg
Potassium 255 mg
Total Carbohydrate 15 g
Dietary Fiber 7 g
Sugars 1 g
Protein 4 g
Phosphorus 90 mg

Celery Root Purée

2 pounds celery root or celeriac, cut into quarters or eighths and peeled

2 cloves garlic

1/2 teaspoon fine sea salt

1/4 teaspoon freshly ground black pepper

1/2 cup skim milk

1/4 cup chopped flat Italian parsley

Celery Root Purée is a great alternative to mashed potatoes and a wonderful side dish to serve at any dinner party! This ugly, brown knob found in the produce department that has great fresh flavor!

SERVES 4 | SERVING SIZE 1/4 recipe
EXCHANGES 1 Starch

1. Place celery root, garlic, salt, and pepper in a 4–quart saucepan and cover with water. Bring to a boil and cook until tender, about 15 minutes (similar to mashed potatoes).

2. Drain and mash with a large fork or potato masher. Stir in milk and parsley.

Cook's Tips

PLACE IN SMALL RAMEKINS AND HEAT IN THE OVEN AT SERVING TIME. SERVE INSTEAD OF POTATOES, RICE, OR PASTA.

Calories 65
  Calories from Fat 0
Total Fat 0 g
  Saturated Fat 0 g
  Trans Fat 0.0 g
Cholesterol 0 mg
Sodium 430 mg
Potassium 400 mg
Total Carbohydrate 14 g
  Dietary Fiber 2 g
  Sugars 4 g
Protein 3 g
Phosphorus 165 mg

Pollo alla Romana (Chicken Roman Style)

2 tablespoons extra virgin olive oil

1 chicken (about 5 pounds), cut into 8 pieces: 2 wings, 2 legs, 2 thighs, 2 breasts (cut in half)

1 onion, cut into fine dice (about 1 cup)

1/2 teaspoon fine sea salt

1/2 teaspoon freshly ground black pepper

1 cup dry white wine, such as Orvieto or Pinot Grigio

2 large red bell peppers, cut into 1/2-inch-wide strips

2 cups canned crushed tomatoes

Crushed red pepper (optional)

This is a recipe from a cooking class I attended in the Trastevere section of Rome. It is a great example of the simplicity of true Italian cooking. This dish is easy to double for a crowd. You can also transfer to a crockpot once browning is done.

SERVES 9 | SERVING SIZE 1/9 recipe | **EXCHANGES** 2 Vegetable, 4 Lean Meat, 1 Fat

1. Place olive oil in pan large enough to hold all chicken pieces in single layer. Add chicken and brown first side. Turn and brown second side and add onion to pan surface. Once chicken is browned on second side, add salt, pepper, wine, bell peppers, and tomatoes. Cover and cook on low 1 hour or until chicken is tender.

2. Optional crushed red pepper can be added at the table.

Calories 275
Calories from Fat 100
Total Fat 11.0 g
Saturated Fat 2.6 g
Trans Fat 0.0 g
Cholesterol 95 mg
Sodium 295 mg
Potassium 545 mg
Total Carbohydrate 9 g
Dietary Fiber 2 g
Sugars 5 g
Protein 32 g
Phosphorus 245 mg

ITALIAN NIGHT

Porchetta (Pork Stuffed with Arugula, Prosciutto, & Mushrooms in White Wine Garlic Sauce)

1 center-cut pork roast (about 3 pounds)

1/2 teaspoon fine sea salt

1/2 teaspoon freshly ground black pepper

6 ounces fresh arugula

4 ounces prosciutto, thinly sliced

5 ounces cremini mushrooms, thinly sliced

2 tablespoons extra virgin olive oil

4 cloves garlic, minced

2 cups dry white Italian wine, such as Pinot Grigio or Orvieto

In Italy, you will find porchetta with many variations, depending on the place you are visiting. Everyone puts their signature on their "roast pork." Feel free to vary my recipe by using it as a guideline with your favorite ingredients.

SERVES 12 | **SERVING SIZE** 1/12 recipe | **EXCHANGES** 3 Lean Meat, 1 1/2 Fat

1. Butterfly pork roast. Pound to even thickness, sprinkle with sea salt and pepper. Top with layers of arugula, prosciutto, and sliced mushrooms. Roll tightly and tie at 2-inch intervals.

2. Place olive oil in large sauté pan and heat. Add the Porchetta. Sear meat on all sides. Add garlic. Cook until fragrant. Deglaze pan with 2 cups white wine. Cover and simmer 20–30 minutes until pork is done, when inside temperature reaches 160°F.

3. Slice into rounds and serve with plenty of juices.

Calories 210
Calories from Fat 100
Total Fat 11.0 g
Saturated Fat 3.2 g
Trans Fat 0.0 g
Cholesterol 65 mg
Sodium 305 mg
Potassium 415 mg
Total Carbohydrate 2 g
Dietary Fiber 0 g
Sugars 1 g
Protein 24 g
Phosphorus 210 mg

Risotto with Chicken & Porcini Mushrooms

1 1/2 cups dry white wine

4 cups low-sodium chicken or mushroom stock

1 cup dried porcini mushrooms, rehydrated*

1 tablespoon extra virgin olive oil

8 ounces boneless, skinless chicken breast, cut into 1/2-inch dice

1 cup onion, chopped

2 cups carnaroli or arborio rice, checked over for imperfect grains

1/2 teaspoon fine sea salt

1/2 teaspoon freshly ground pepper

1/2 cup freshly grated Parmigiano-Reggiano cheese

2 tablespoons finely minced Italian parsley

The key to good risotto is the slow absorption of the hot liquid, which can take 20–40 minutes. Risotto is worth the wait so don't rush the process. The slow cooking is what provides the creaminess of the dish.

SERVES 6 | SERVING SIZE 1/6 recipe
EXCHANGES 3 Starch, 1 Vegetable, 1 Lean Meat, 1/2 Fat

1. *To rehydrate the mushrooms: bring wine and stock to a boil in a 4–quart saucepan. Reduce heat to a simmer. Add porcini mushrooms and simmer 5 minutes. Drain this mixture through a coffee filter, reserving the stock/wine mixture. Remove porcini and chop into bite–size pieces. Place stock/wine back in pan and simmer. (The purpose of straining is to clear the liquid of any dirt that might have been on the porcini.)

2. Using a heavy 5–quart saucepan or chef's pan, add the olive oil and add chicken and onion. Sauté until chicken is golden and onion starts to soften. Add rice, salt, and pepper and coat rice grains with olive oil mixture. Add stock mixture 1 cup at a time and stir until each addition of liquid is absorbed. This takes time and patience. After last addition of stock is absorbed, add Parmigiano–Reggiano. When all of the stock is absorbed, which can take anywhere from 20–40 minutes, and rice grains are creamy, you can add the parsley and porcini.

Calories 340
  Calories from Fat 55
Total Fat 6.0 g
  Saturated Fat 2.1 g
  Trans Fat 0.0 g
Cholesterol 30 mg
Sodium 320 mg
Potassium 380 mg
Total Carbohydrate 52 g
  Dietary Fiber 3 g
  Sugars 2 g
Protein 17 g
Phosphorus 210 mg

Rosemary Vincotto Chicken

2 tablespoons extra virgin olive oil

1 teaspoon fine sea salt

1/2 teaspoon freshly ground black pepper

1 chicken (about 5 pounds), cut into 9 pieces, skin removed

2 garlic cloves, sliced thinly

2 sprigs fresh rosemary

2 tablespoons fig vincotto

1/4 dry white wine, preferably Italian, such as Orvieto or Pinot Grigio

1/2 cup low-sodium chicken stock

1/4 cup chopped Italian parsley

Vincotto is cooked grape must that ends up being a very sweet condiment for cooking. In this dish I used a fig vincotto, but you can use any vincotto that you can get your hands on. It's a wonderful addition to your pantry.

SERVES 9 | SERVING SIZE 1/9 recipe | **EXCHANGES** 4 Lean Meat, 1 Fat

1. Place extra virgin olive oil in a sauté pan large enough to hold the chicken parts in a single layer. Season chicken on both sides with salt and pepper. Heat pan to medium and add chicken to pan. Brown chicken on first side. Turn over and brown second side.

2. While chicken is browning on second side, add garlic and rosemary to the pan surface and continue to brown chicken. Once chicken is completely brown, add vincotto, wine, and chicken stock. Bring to a boil and then turn down to medium. Cover and cook 20 minutes. Add parsley and cook another 20–30 minutes until chicken is cooked to 165°F.

Calories 240
  Calories from Fat 100
Total Fat 11.0 g
  Saturated Fat 2.6 g
  Trans Fat 0.0 g
Cholesterol 95 mg
Sodium 360 mg
Potassium 285 mg
Total Carbohydrate 2 g
  Dietary Fiber 0 g
  Sugars 1 g
Protein 31 g
Phosphorus 210 mg

Spinaci Alla Fiorentina

2 bags (10 ounces each) baby
  spinach

1/2 cup pignoli nuts (pine nuts)

3 cloves garlic, finely minced

1/4 teaspoon fine sea salt

1/8 teaspoon freshly ground black
  pepper

1/2 cup raisins

2 teaspoons extra virgin olive oil

Another one of the wonderful recipes that I have gotten from a cooking school in Italy. This is a dish that is worthy of the best olive oil you have in your kitchen, since it "finishes" the dish.

SERVES 6 | **SERVING SIZE** 1/6 recipe | **EXCHANGES** 1/2 Fruit, 1 Vegetable, 2 Fat

1. Wash spinach and drain in colander.

2. To toast nuts: Place nuts in dry skillet. Heat pan and shake nuts occasionally until they begin to brown. Remove from pan and let cool on dinner plate to stop cooking process.

3. Place spinach and garlic in large sauté pan. Cook with the water that clings to spinach. Season with salt and pepper. Add pignoli and raisins. Cook until dish is hot and well blended.

4. Drizzle with good-quality extra virgin olive oil.

Cook's Tips

ADDITIONAL TOASTED NUTS WILL KEEP IN AN AIRTIGHT CONTAINER IN THE REFRIGERATOR FOR WEEKS.

Calories 150
  Calories from Fat 90
Total Fat 10.0 g
  Saturated Fat 0.8 g
  Trans Fat 0.0 g
Cholesterol 0 mg
Sodium 175 mg
Potassium 690 mg
Total Carbohydrate 15 g
  Dietary Fiber 3 g
  Sugars 8 g
Protein 5 g
Phosphorus 125 mg

ITALIAN
NIGHT

Traditional Italian-Style Meatballs

3 garlic cloves, minced

1 small onion, minced

1/2 cup egg substitute

1 tablespoon chopped fresh basil

1/2 cup chopped fresh parsley

2 tablespoons freshly grated Parmesan cheese

1/2 teaspoon fine sea salt

1/2 teaspoon ground black pepper

1/2 cup Italian-style breadcrumbs

1/4 cup low-sodium beef broth or red wine

1 1/2 pounds extra-lean (95%) ground beef

It would be rare to see spaghetti and meatballs served in Italy. That is more of an Italian-American dish. Rolled into 1-inch meatballs and placed in Mushroom Sherry Sauce (page 167), you will have a great cocktail appetizer. Or simmer in Quick Marinara Sauce (see page 125) for a more traditional dish. You can also use this recipe to make a delicious meatloaf, for a change of pace.

SERVES 21 | SERVING SIZE 1 meatball **| EXCHANGES** 1 Lean Meat

1. Preheat oven to 425°F; use convection if you have it.

2. Place all ingredients except the beef in a large bowl. Mix well and then add the beef and gently mix. Roll dough into a log and cut into 21 pieces. Roll into balls. If the mixture does not hold together, add 1/4 cup additional breadcrumbs.

3. Place the meatballs on a parchment-lined baking sheet and bake in a very hot oven to brown the outside.

4. Place in your favorite sauce or freeze until needed.

Cook's Tips

YOU DON'T WANT TO OVER MIX OR YOUR MEATBALLS WILL BE TOUGH. THAT IS WHY I LIKE TO THE MIX EVERYTHING BUT THE MEAT TOGETHER BEFORE ADDING THE MEAT.

Calories 60
Calories from Fat 20
Total Fat 2.0 g
Saturated Fat 0.9 g
Trans Fat 0.0 g
Cholesterol 20 mg
Sodium 135 mg
Potassium 135 mg
Total Carbohydrate 3 g
Dietary Fiber 0 g
Sugars 0 g
Protein 8 g
Phosphorus 70 mg

ITALIAN
NIGHT

Veal Milanese

1 cup Italian-seasoned breadcrumbs

1 teaspoon of your custom herb blend or Italian Seasoning

1/8 teaspoon fine sea salt

1/2 teaspoon ground black pepper

3/4 cup egg substitute

2 tablespoons extra virgin olive oil

16 ounces scaloppini of veal, pork, chicken, or turkey

"Scaloppini" is a very thin cut of veal. While it's traditionally served with veal, I find that pork, chicken, and turkey are all delicious prepared this way. If the scaloppini cut is not available, just pound your choice of protein to 1/4 inch thick using a flat meat pounder with the meat placed between two sheets of parchment.

This dish is classically served with a Tre Colore Salad with Vinaigrette (see page 24) on top of the warm veal.

SERVES 4 | SERVING SIZE 1/4 recipe | EXCHANGES 1 Starch, 4 Lean Meat, 1 Fat

1. Mix the breadcrumbs, herb blend, salt, pepper, and cheese together in a pie plate.

2. Scramble the egg in a pie plate.

3. Dip the cutlets in the egg and then the breadcrumbs. You might have extra breadcrumbs and egg left over. You should discard this. The crumbs will adhere to the cutlets better if you do this and refrigerate for a few minutes or early in the day.

4. Heat the olive oil in a nonstick sauté pan and cook each cutlet until golden brown on each side.

Calories 300
 Calories from Fat 115
Total Fat 13.0 g
 Saturated Fat 2.6 g
 Trans Fat 0.0 g
Cholesterol 90 mg
Sodium 460 mg
Potassium 355 mg
Total Carbohydrate 14 g
 Dietary Fiber 1 g
 Sugars 1 g
Protein 30 g
Phosphorus 220 mg

Veal Ragu for Pasta

3 tablespoons extra virgin olive oil

1 large onion, chopped (about 1 cup)

3 pounds lean veal shoulder, cut into chunks

12 fresh plum tomatoes, cut into large chunks

1 (28-ounce) can crushed tomatoes

1 (16-ounce) can diced tomatoes

1 cup fresh basil, chopped

This recipe was inspired by a wonderful chef, Rocco Cartia, who visited my home and taught a cooking class to many of my Italian food and wine friends. Everyone just loved it. This would be a good example of a "Sunday Sauce" in Italy.

SERVES 12 | **SERVING SIZE** 1/12 recipe | **EXCHANGES** 2 Vegetable, 3 Lean Meat, 1 Fat

1. Place olive oil in large saucepan. Add onion and cook until translucent.

2. Add veal cubes in single layer and brown on all sides. Add tomatoes and cook at low boil for at least an hour.

3. Stir in basil. If serving with pasta, add cooked pasta to sauce.

Calories 225
Calories from Fat 80
Total Fat 9.0 g
Saturated Fat 1.9 g
Trans Fat 0.0 g
Cholesterol 90 mg
Sodium 215 mg
Potassium 715 mg
Total Carbohydrate 11 g
Dietary Fiber 3 g
Sugars 6 g
Protein 26 g
Phosphorus 240 mg

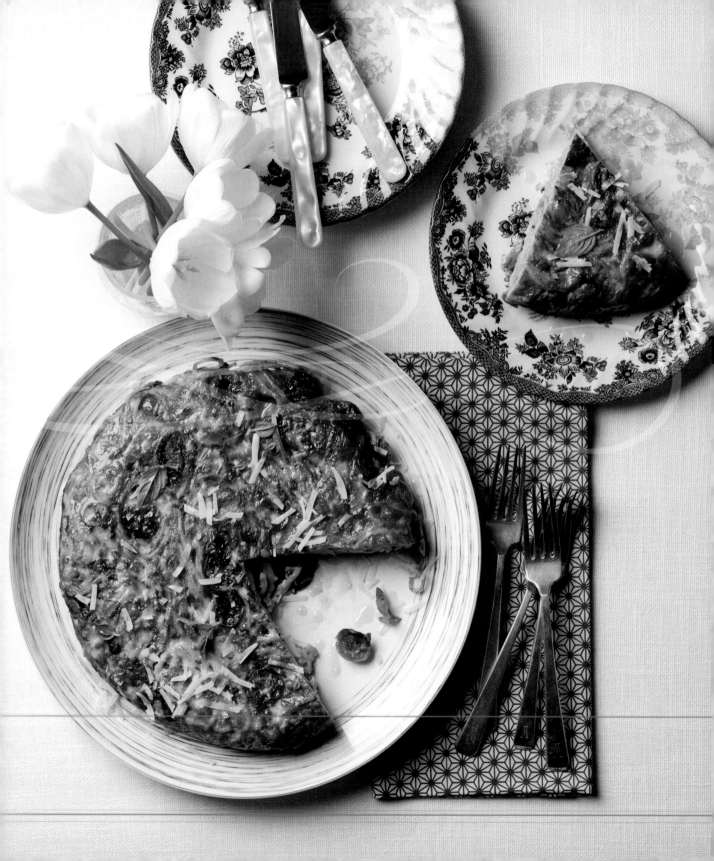

MEATLESS MONDAYS

Baby Eggplant Fans with White Beans & Roasted Red Pepper Dressing

3 tablespoons extra virgin olive oil, plus 1 teaspoon for dressing

8 large cloves garlic, sliced lengthwise

1 lemon, juiced

Fresh rosemary

15 ounces canned white beans, drained and rinsed well

3/4 teaspoon fine sea salt

Freshly ground pepper, to taste

4 baby eggplants, individual serving size

4 Roasted Peppers (See page 20), roasted

SERVES 4 | SERVING SIZE 1/4 recipe | **EXCHANGES** 1 Starch, 3 Vegetable, 2 1/2 Fat

1. Preheat oven to 425°F.

2. Place 3 tablespoons olive oil in small saucepan. Heat and then add sliced garlic. Watch carefully and cook until golden. Remove garlic from oil with slotted spoon.

3. Mix the warm olive oil with lemon juice, rosemary, and beans. Add salt and pepper to taste. Set aside. (This step can be done several hours ahead.)

4. Slice eggplant into fans. Sprinkle salt between slices. Place on parchment-lined baking sheet and roast until eggplant is tender, approximately 20 minutes (this will vary depending on eggplant size and type).

5. Place eggplant on individual serving dish and fill with some of the bean salad, allowing beans to spill out on plate.

6. Place roasted peppers in food processor and process until smooth. Add a drop of balsamic vinegar and 1 teaspoon extra virgin olive oil. Process again. Drizzle over eggplant and beans. Garnish with fresh rosemary sprigs and freshly ground pepper.

Calories 270
Calories from Fat 110
Total Fat 12.0 g
Saturated Fat 1.7 g
Trans Fat 0.0 g
Cholesterol 0 mg
Sodium 515 mg
Potassium 715 mg
Total Carbohydrate 34 g
Dietary Fiber 10 g
Sugars 10 g
Protein 8 g
Phosphorus 145 mg

MEATLESS MONDAYS

1 pound pasta (shape of your choice)

2 tablespoons extra virgin olive oil

3 garlic cloves, minced

3 cups fresh vegetables, cut into bite-sized pieces (such as broccoli, red bell pepper, zucchini, onion, carrots, green beans, eggplant, or peas)

2 1/4 cups chicken or vegetable stock (divided use)

Few drops balsamic vinegar

1/2 cup fresh basil leaves, chiffonade, or 2 tablespoons dried basil

1/2 cup fresh Italian parsley, chopped, or 2 tablespoons dried parsley

1/4 cup fresh oregano, chopped, or 1 tablespoon dried oregano

1/2 cup freshly grated Parmigiano-Reggiano cheese

1 cup dry white wine

Additional chopped fresh herbs, for garnish

Have fun creating your own signature dish by using whatever veggies you like.

SERVES 8 | SERVING SIZE 1/8 recipe | EXCHANGES 2 1/2 Starch, 1 Vegetable, 1 Fat

1. Cook pasta in 8 quarts of boiling salted water. Drain and set aside.

2. Place olive oil and garlic in large sauté pan. Cook until garlic is fragrant. Do not brown.

3. Add fresh vegetables and approximately 1/4 cup stock and sauté until crisp-tender.

4. Sprinkle with balsamic vinegar and garnish with fresh herbs and Parmigiano-Reggiano cheese.

5. Add remaining stock and wine and bring to a boil. Immediately turn down heat to low. Add pasta and herbs and toss well.

Calories 295
Calories from Fat 55
Total Fat 6.0 g
Saturated Fat 1.7 g
Trans Fat 0.0 g
Cholesterol 5 mg
Sodium 325 mg
Potassium 240 mg
Total Carbohydrate 45 g
Dietary Fiber 7 g
Sugars 3 g
Protein 12 g
Phosphorus 175 mg

MEATLESS
MONDAYS

Escarole Pie

SOFT PIZZA DOUGH

1 cup 00 flour (found in Italian specialty markets)

1 cup all-purpose flour

1 teaspoon yeast

1/2 teaspoon fine sea salt

1/2 cup water at 110–120°F (use an instant-read meat thermometer)

ESCAROLE MIXTURE

2 pounds fresh escarole

1 tablespoon extra virgin olive oil

4 cloves garlic, minced

Pinch crushed red pepper

1 cup diced onion (about 5 ounces or 1/2 large)

1 teaspoon Salt & Pepper Blend (page viii)

1/4 cup grated Pecorino cheese

1/2 cup part-skim shredded mozzarella

nonstick cooking spray

1 egg white, scrambled

Calories 185
Calories from Fat 35
Total Fat 4.0 g
Saturated Fat 1.7 g
Trans Fat 0.0 g
Cholesterol 5 mg
Sodium 470 mg
Potassium 400 mg
Total Carbohydrate 30 g
Dietary Fiber 4 g
Sugars 1 g
Protein 7 g
Phosphorus 120 mg

This is a traditional Italian holiday dish, but I think it also makes a wonderful meatless meal with sliced tomatoes and basil or a Roasted Beet Salad (page 60) and a glass of crisp dry white wine, such as Orvieto.

SERVES 8 | SERVING SIZE 1/8 recipe | EXCHANGES 1 1/2 Starch, 1 Vegetable, 1 Fat

1. Place all pizza dough ingredients in food processor fitted with steel blade. Process until mixture forms a ball. If it is too grainy, you can add more water, 1 tablespoon at time, until ball forms.

2. Remove dough from food processor and place in large bowl that has been rubbed with extra virgin olive oil. Turn ball to coat. Cover with plastic wrap and let rise in warm place until doubled in size, at least 1 hour.

3. While pizza dough is rising, prepare escarole mixture. Wash and dry escarole. Cut into small pieces.

4. Place olive oil in large sauté pan. Add garlic, red pepper, and onion and cook on medium until onion is translucent. Add escarole and Salt & Pepper Blend and sauté until escarole wilts to less than half. Cool. Add cheese to escarole. Mix well.

5. Roll pizza dough out as thinly as possible so that it is several inches larger than a 9–inch pie plate. Spray pie plate with nonstick cooking spray. Place dough in pie plate. Fill with cooled escarole mixture.

6. Fold pizza dough over the escarole mixture so that it overlaps all the way around the pie plate. It will not cover entire mixture. Brush crust with egg white.

7. Preheat oven to 375°F convection oven or 400°F traditional oven. Bake the escarole pie about 35–45 minutes or until crust is golden brown.

Cook's Tips

00 FLOUR IS IMPORTED FROM ITALY AND IS A MORE FINELY GROUND FLOUR, WHICH YIELDS A MORE "FRIENDLY," EASY-TO-WORK WITH DOUGH.

Fava Purée

1 small onion, about 1/2 cup finely diced

1 small potato, about 1 cup finely diced

2 pounds dried, skinless fava beans

1/4 cup extra virgin olive oil

1 teaspoon fine sea salt

1/2 teaspoon freshly ground black pepper

Fava are also called broad beans. They are a wonderful spring vegetable, but this recipe calls for dried fava. In Italy, they are known as fave and are a specialty of the region of Puglia, which is the heel of the boot. This recipe is from my friend Val, whose mother was from Puglia. I've had this dish served with sautéed chicory or kale on top and Val serves it with broccoli rabe on the side. You decide!

SERVES 12 | **SERVING SIZE** 1/12 recipe | **EXCHANGES** 2 1/2 Starch, 2 Lean Meat

1. Place diced onion and potato on bottom of medium saucepan. Pour fava over onion and potato. Cover fava with water.

2. Bring pan to a boil. Reduce heat, cover, and simmer until fava are tender and the water has been absorbed. Add additional water if needed until fava are tender. Allow to cool a few minutes.

3. Purée contents with a hand blender to consistency of mashed potatoes. Blend in extra virgin olive oil. Add salt and pepper.

Cook's Tips

IF FAVA ARE A LITTLE TOO WATERY, ADD IN A FEW CUBED PIECES OF DAY-OLD BREAD TO TIGHTEN.

CAN BE SERVED AS A VEGETARIAN ENTRÉE ALONGSIDE A DARK GREEN VEGGIE, SUCH AS BROCCOLI RABE, OR AS A SIDE DISH WITH MOST MEATS (SAUSAGE IS GREAT). ALSO GREAT AS A SPREAD ON BRUSCHETTA.

Calories 280
  Calories from Fat 45
Total Fat 5.0 g
  Saturated Fat 0.8 g
  Trans Fat 0.0 g
Cholesterol 0 mg
Sodium 210 mg
Potassium 630 mg
Total Carbohydrate 44 g
  Dietary Fiber 12 g
  Sugars 4 g
Protein 16 g
Phosphorus 270 mg

Tomato Basil Frittata

3 large eggs

6 egg whites

1/2 teaspoon fine sea salt

1/2 teaspoon ground black pepper
or crushed red pepper flakes

1 cup basil leaves, chopped

1/4 cup oregano leaves, chopped

1/2 cup grated Parmigiano-
Reggiano cheese

3 cups sliced cherry or grape
tomatoes

1/2 pound cooked spaghetti

Extra virgin olive oil pan spray

Additional Parmigiano for garnish
(optional)

This frittata makes great use of leftover spaghetti. It has all of our favorite things like tomatoes, basil, and Parmigiano-Reggiano, and the extra protein from eggs. Use a good-quality egg that is lower in saturated fat. If you like spicy dishes, use the crushed red pepper flakes instead of the black pepper. Serve with a salad or fruit and you'll have a high-protein, quick, and easy meal. You can also add vegetables such as asparagus or broccoli to this dish.

SERVES 6 | SERVING SIZE 1/6 frittata
EXCHANGES 1 Starch, 1 Vegetable, 1 Lean Meat, 1/2 Fat

1. Whisk eggs and egg whites in large mixing bowl. Add salt, pepper, basil, oregano, and Parmigiano. Mix well. Add tomatoes and spaghetti and mix well.

2. Spray sauté pan lightly with extra virgin olive oil spray. Add egg mixture. Cook on medium–high heat about 7 minutes until the bottom is golden. Place dinner plate on top of sauté pan. Turn the pan over so that the frittata is bottom side up on the plate. Slide frittata back into the sauté pan and cook until the second side is golden, about 4–5 minutes. You can cover it to cook it more quickly.

3. Once done, sprinkle with grated cheese. Cover to melt cheese and keep warm. Cut into wedges and serve.

Calories 160
  Calories from Fat 45
Total Fat 5.0 g
  Saturated Fat 2.3 g
  Trans Fat 0.0 g
Cholesterol 100 mg
Sodium 335 mg
Potassium 395 mg
Total Carbohydrate 17 g
  Dietary Fiber 3 g
  Sugars 3 g
Protein 12 g
Phosphorus 155 mg

**MEATLESS
MONDAYS**

Orzo & Lentil Salad with Broccoli & Sun-Dried Tomatoes

1 cup uncooked lentils, preferably French or small dark green

16 ounces uncooked orzo (rice shaped pasta), or the pasta shape of your choice

1 head broccoli, broken into florets

1 cup sun-dried tomatoes (not purchased in oil)

3 tablespoons white balsamic vinegar

2 cloves garlic, minced

1 tablespoon fresh oregano, chopped

1/2 cup fresh basil leaves, torn

1/2 teaspoon fine sea salt

1/4 teaspoon freshly ground black pepper

1/3 cup extra virgin olive oil

3/4 cup crumbled fat-free feta cheese

1/2 cup toasted pignoli nuts (pine nuts)

Additional herbs for garnish (basil)

SERVES 8 | SERVING SIZE 1/8 recipe
EXCHANGES 3 1/2 Starch, 1 Vegetable, 1 Lean Meat, 2 1/2 Fat

1. Cook lentils in 3 cups water until tender, approximately 20 minutes.

2. Cook orzo according to package directions, approximately 9 minutes. Add broccoli during last 5 minutes of cooking time. Drain.

3. To rehydrate (soften) sun-dried tomatoes: Bring a small pot of water to a boil and add tomatoes. Turn heat off and let sit while orzo and lentils are cooking. Drain.

4. Place balsamic in bowl. Add garlic, oregano, basil, sea salt, and pepper. Slowly whisk in olive oil. Set aside.

5. Mix orzo, lentils, sun-dried tomatoes, cheese, and nuts together. Add dressing. Taste and adjust seasonings. Can be made a day or two ahead and kept refrigerated. Garnish with fresh herbs before serving.

Cook's Tips

GREAT FOR PICNICS, MAKE-AHEAD MEALS, OR BROWN BAG LUNCHES.

Calories 465
Calories from Fat 145
Total Fat 16.0 g
Saturated Fat 1.9 g
Trans Fat 0.0 g
Cholesterol 0 mg
Sodium 515 mg
Potassium 780 mg
Total Carbohydrate 63 g
Dietary Fiber 10 g
Sugars 12 g
Protein 19 g
Phosphorus 355 mg

Fresh Vegetable Stew with Chickpeas

1 medium-to-large zucchini

2 large carrots

1 head cauliflower, broken into small florets

2 (10-ounce) cans chickpeas, drained and rinsed (or any beans you like)

2 tablespoons extra virgin olive oil

3 cloves garlic, minced

2 teaspoons Italian seasoning blend

3 bay leaves

28 ounces no-salt-added diced tomatoes

1 teaspoon Salt & Pepper Blend (page viii)

Use this recipe as a guideline for creating many delicious vegetable stews. Substitute your favorite vegetables and beans for variety.

SERVES 6 | **SERVING SIZE** 1/6 recipe | **EXCHANGES** 1 Starch, 2 Vegetable, 1 1/2 Fat

1. Thinly slice zucchini into rounds. Cut carrots into 2-inch lengths. Break cauliflower into small florets. Drain chickpeas in a colander and rinse well.

2. Place the olive oil in the skillet. Add garlic and cook until it becomes fragrant. Add carrots and cauliflower and cook until they begin to soften, about 5 minutes. Add zucchini and mix well. Clear a space in the bottom of the pan and add the Italian seasoning and bay leaves. Cook 1 minute until the seasoning becomes fragrant. Add chickpeas, tomatoes, and Salt & Pepper Blend and cook for 10 minutes.

Cook's Tips

DRAINING CANNED BEANS HELPS TO REMOVE ANY PRESERVATIVES AND SOME OF THE GAS.

REMOVE THE BAY LEAVES BEFORE SERVING. THEY ARE SHARP AND CAN CAUSE INJURY IF SWALLOWED.

Calories 190
  Calories from Fat 55
Total Fat 6.0 g
  Saturated Fat 0.9 g
  Trans Fat 0.0 g
Cholesterol 0 mg
Sodium 390 mg
Potassium 835 mg
Total Carbohydrate 29 g
  Dietary Fiber 8 g
  Sugars 9 g
Protein 8 g
Phosphorus 180 mg

Orzo Salad with Roasted Eggplant, Zucchini & Red Pepper

1 cup uncooked lentils, preferably French or small dark green

16 ounces uncooked whole-wheat orzo (rice-shaped pasta), or the pasta shape of your choice

1/4 cup red wine vinegar

2 cloves garlic, minced

1 tablespoon fresh oregano, chopped

1/2 cup fresh basil leaves, torn

1/2 teaspoon fine sea salt

1/4 teaspoon freshly ground black pepper

1/3 cup extra virgin olive oil

4 cups Grilled Vegetables (see page 11)

3/4 cup freshly grated Grana Padano cheese

Additional herbs for garnish

This salad is a great way to use leftover roasted or grilled veggies. Grana Padano cheese is lower in fat as it is made from part-skim milk.

SERVES 8 | SERVING SIZE 1/8 recipe
EXCHANGES 3 1/2 Starch, 1 Vegetable, 1 Lean Meat, 1 1/2 Fat

1. Cook lentils in 3 cups water until tender, approximately 20 minutes. Drain. Place in large bowl.

2. Cook orzo according to package directions, approximately 9 minutes. Drain. Place in large bowl with lentils.

3. Place vinegar in separate bowl. Add garlic, oregano, basil, sea salt, and pepper. Slowly whisk in olive oil. Set aside.

4. Mix orzo, lentils, veggies, and cheese together. Add dressing. Taste and adjust seasonings. Can be made a day or two ahead and kept refrigerated. Garnish with fresh herbs before serving.

Cook's Tips

GREET FOR PICNICS, MAKE–AHEAD MEALS OR BROWN BAG LUNCHES.

Calories 410
Calories from Fat 115
Total Fat 13.0 g
Saturated Fat 3.3 g
Trans Fat 0.0 g
Cholesterol 10 mg
Sodium 215 mg
Potassium 515 mg
Total Carbohydrate 61 g
Dietary Fiber 11 g
Sugars 6 g
Protein 18 g
Phosphorus 350 mg

Pasta with Cauliflower Sauce

8 ounces mafaldine pasta (thin lasagna) or your favorite shape

2 tablespoons extra virgin olive oil

1 medium head cauliflower, cut into florets

2 large garlic cloves, crushed and peeled

2 cups cannellini beans, drained and rinsed well

2 cups vegetable stock

1 cup grape tomatoes, cut in half

1/2 cup chopped Italian parsley

2 1/2 ounces aged Asiago cheese, coarsely grated

Pinch of crushed red pepper (optional)

SERVES 4 | SERVING SIZE 1/6 recipe | **EXCHANGES** 2 1/2 Starch, 1 Vegetable, 1 Med-Fat Meat, 1/2 Fat

1. Cook pasta to al dente stage. While pasta is cooking, prepare the sauce.

2. Place olive oil in pan. Turn pan to medium–high heat. Add cauliflower and garlic. Cook until garlic is fragrant, about 2–3 minutes.

3. Add beans and stock and cover. Cook until cauliflower is fork tender. Add tomatœs. Toss well and cover. Turn heat to low.

4. Drain pasta and add to pan with sauce. Toss well. Add parsley and cheese. Add crushed red pepper, if desired.

Calories 325
Calories from Fat 80
Total Fat 9.0 g
Saturated Fat 3.3 g
Trans Fat 0.0 g
Cholesterol 10 mg
Sodium 515 mg
Potassium 610 mg
Total Carbohydrate 47 g
Dietary Fiber 6 g
Sugars 5 g
Protein 14 g
Phosphorus 250 mg

MEATLESS MONDAYS

Pasta with Lemon, Pepper & Fresh Herbs

2 cloves garlic, peeled and sliced thin

1/3 cup extra virgin olive oil

1/2 teaspoon fine sea salt

1/4 teaspoon freshly ground black pepper

1/2 cup fresh lemon juice, about 3 lemons (room temperature)

1 pound linguine, cooked al dente

1/2 cup roughly chopped fresh herbs (such as Italian parsley, basil, or chives)

The freshness of the lemon makes this dish perfect for a warm summer evening. To add variety to your meal plan, try preparing this dish with alternative pastas, such as those made with rice, farro, spelt, or corn.

SERVES 8 | SERVING SIZE 1 cup | **EXCHANGES** 3 Starch, 1 1/2 Fat

1. Place garlic and olive oil in small saucepan. Cook until garlic is light to golden brown. Immediately remove from heat and transfer to heatproof bowl.

2. Add sea salt and pepper. Add lemon juice. Whisk together until creamy. Pour over cooked, hot pasta and toss well.

3. Garnish with fresh herbs and additional lemon slices, if desired.

Cook's Tips

CAN ALSO BE SERVED ROOM TEMPERATURE, WHICH MAKES IT GREAT FOR BUFFETS.

Calories 305
Calories from Fat 90
Total Fat 10.0 g
Saturated Fat 1.5 g
Trans Fat 0.0 g
Cholesterol 0 mg
Sodium 155 mg
Potassium 90 mg
Total Carbohydrate 45 g
Dietary Fiber 3 g
Sugars 1 g
Protein 8 g
Phosphorus 85 mg

Penne alla Vodka

1 pound whole-wheat penne pasta, cooked al dente according to package directions

1/4 cup extra virgin olive oil

10 cloves garlic, crushed and peeled

1 (28-ounce) can San Marzano tomatoes

1/2 teaspoon fine sea salt

1/4 teaspoon crushed red pepper flakes

1/4 cup vodka

1/2 cup evaporated skim milk

2/3 cup freshly grated Parmigiano-Reggiano cheese

This dish is one of America's favorites and can be made with any number of high-fat ingredients such as butter and cream, but I have lightened it up by using extra virgin olive oil and evaporated skim milk. The evaporated milk is a little creamier than regular nonfat milk.

SERVES 8 | **SERVING SIZE** 1/8 recipe | **EXCHANGES** 3 Starch, 1 Vegetable, 1 1/2 Fat

1. While pasta is cooking, heat the olive oil in a large skillet. Add the garlic and cook until lightly browned.

2. Add the tomatoes. Bring to a boil. Season with salt and crushed red pepper. Cook 2 minutes.

3. Add vodka and simmer a couple of minutes. Add milk. Add the pasta and toss. Add the cheese and toss to blend. Serve immediately.

Calories 345
  Calories from Fat 90
Total Fat 10.0 g
  Saturated Fat 2.5 g
  Trans Fat 0.0 g
Cholesterol 5 mg
Sodium 360 mg
Potassium 310 mg
Total Carbohydrate 52 g
  Dietary Fiber 7 g
  Sugars 6 g
Protein 11 g
Phosphorus 205 mg

MEATLESS MONDAYS

Polenta with Asparagus & Cremini Mushrooms

6 cups vegetable stock

2 cloves garlic, minced

1/2 teaspoon fine sea salt

2 cups uncooked polenta or yellow cornmeal

1 teaspoon extra virgin olive oil

1 pound asparagus, thin, if available

10 ounces cremini mushrooms, sliced

1 cup low-sodium vegetable stock (divided use)

1/2 teaspoon freshly ground black pepper

1/2 cup chopped fresh herbs, such as basil, marjoram, and Italian parsley

SERVES 8 | SERVING SIZE 1/8 recipe | EXCHANGES 2 Starch, 1 Vegetable

1. In a heavy saucepan, bring stock to a boil and add garlic and salt. Add the cornmeal, stirring constantly with a spoon. Cook until thick, approximately 10–15 minutes.

2. While polenta is cooking, sauté the vegetables. Place olive oil in large sauté pan. Add asparagus. Sauté until asparagus is crisp-tender. Remove.

3. Add mushrooms to pan. Sauté and add stock as necessary to continue to sauté. Heat to boil and add remaining stock. Cook 3–5 minutes. Turn pan to low and keep warm. Return asparagus to pan. Season with pepper.

4. Place a scoop of polenta in the center of the plate. Top with vegetables and fresh herbs.

Calories 165
  Calories from Fat 10
Total Fat 1.0 g
  Saturated Fat 0.2 g
  Trans Fat 0.0 g
Cholesterol 0 mg
Sodium 280 mg
Potassium 405 mg
Total Carbohydrate 33 g
  Dietary Fiber 4 g
  Sugars 3 g
Protein 5 g
Phosphorus 165 mg

Polenta with Porcini Mushroom Sauce

2 ounces dried porcini (or any dried mushroom except morels)

2 portobello mushroom caps

1 tablespoon extra virgin olive oil

1 medium onion, chopped

2 cloves garlic, minced

1/2 cup dry red wine

28 ounces low-sodium canned crushed tomatoes

1/2 cup fresh basil leaves

1 tablespoon fresh oregano leaves

1 cup uncooked polenta

Mushrooms make great substitutes for meat with their hearty, earthy, and rich flavor. Portobello mushrooms are often referred to as the vegetarian filet mignon. This sauce is also great over farro or your favorite grain. Pinot noir is a great wine to pair with mushrooms.

SERVES 6 | **SERVING SIZE** 1/6 recipe | **EXCHANGES** 3 Vegetable, 1/2 Fat

1. Bring 2 cups water to a boil. Add porcini, remove from heat, and let sit 3–5 minutes. Drain and save liquid. Chop porcini.

2. Place extra virgin olive oil in 6–quart saucepan. Add onion and garlic. Cook until onion is translucent and garlic is fragrant. (Do not brown the garlic.) Add mushrooms.

3. Add wine and deglaze pan. Add mushroom liquid, tomatoes, basil, and oregano. Simmer for 30 minutes or longer.

4. Bring 4 cups water to a boil. Whisk in 1 cup polenta and cook until thickened, about 10 minutes. Drizzle mushroom sauce over polenta.

Cook's Tips

THIS SAUCE ALSO FREEZES WELL.

YOU CAN ALSO USE THE CROCKPOT ON LOW 8 HOURS OR HIGH FOR 4 HOURS.

THIS SAUCE GOES WELL WITH ANY GRILLED PROTEIN OR PASTA.

Calories 110
Calories from Fat 25
Total Fat 3.0 g
Saturated Fat 0.4 g
Trans Fat 0.0 g
Cholesterol 0 mg
Sodium 10 mg
Potassium 665 mg
Total Carbohydrate 17 g
Dietary Fiber 4 g
Sugars 6 g
Protein 4 g
Phosphorus 105 mg

Ricotta Spinach Pie with Tomato & Goat Cheese

Nonstick olive oil cooking spray

1 tablespoon extra virgin olive oil

1/2 cup chopped onion, about 1 small

3 cups baby spinach

2 large eggs

2 large egg whites

1/2 cup skim milk

1 cup fat-free ricotta

1/2 teaspoon Salt & Pepper Blend (page viii)

8 sheets of phyllo dough, defrosted in the fridge (you won't need a whole package)

3 plum tomatoes, sliced 1/4-inch thick

1/4 cup reduced-fat crumbled goat cheese with garlic and herbs

I love the combination of ricotta, spinach, and tomato, and in this recipe I've been able to combine them to make a "meatless" meal. This would also be great as a brunch item, first course, or prepared in a square pan and cut into small pieces to be served as an appetizer.

SERVES 8 | SERVING SIZE 1 slice | EXCHANGES 1 Starch, 1 Vegetable, 1 Lean Meat, 1/2 Fat

1. Preheat oven to 375°F.

2. Spray a 9-inch pie pan with nonstick cooking spray.

3. Place olive oil in medium sauté pan. Add onion and cook until onion begins to soften. Add spinach and wilt. Turn pan off. Cool.

4. Place eggs, egg whites, milk, ricotta, and Salt & Pepper Blend in a medium mixing bowl. Whisk together until smooth. Add onion and spinach.

5. Lay phyllo out on work surface. Place one sheet in the pie pan. Spray with nonstick cooking spray. Lay second sheet on the first at a different angle. Repeat with each sheet, turning each sheet so that when you are done, there is phyllo overlapping the entire pie pan.

6. Pour in egg mixture. Fold phyllo edge, under each other to create a nice edge. Spray edges with nonstick cooking spray. Top with sliced tomatoes and goat cheese.

7. Bake 35 minutes until middle is set and top begins to brown. Cool at least 10 minutes before cutting.

Calories 160
  Calories from Fat 40
Total Fat 4.5 g
  Saturated Fat 1.1 g
  Trans Fat 0.0 g
Cholesterol 60 mg
Sodium 290 mg
Potassium 300 mg
Total Carbohydrate 20 g
  Dietary Fiber 1 g
  Sugars 3 g
Protein 10 g
Phosphorus 145 mg

MEATLESS MONDAYS

Risotto with Porcini Mushrooms

1 1/2 cups dry white wine

4 cups low-sodium stock, such as vegetable or mushroom

1 cup dried porcini, or any dried mushroom

2 tablespoons extra virgin olive oil

1 cup chopped onion (about 1 medium)

2 cups carnaroli or arborio rice, checked over for imperfect grains

1/2 teaspoon fine sea salt

1/2 teaspoon freshly ground pepper

1/2 cup freshly grated Parmigiano-Reggiano cheese

2 tablespoons finely minced Italian parsley

The key to good risotto is the slow absorption of the hot liquid, which takes anywhere from 20–40 minutes.

SERVES 6 | SERVING SIZE 1/6 recipe | EXCHANGES 3 Starch, 1 Vegetable, 1 Fat

1. Bring wine and stock to a boil in a 4–quart saucepan. Reduce heat and keep at a simmer on stove. Add porcini and let sit 5 minutes. Drain porcini, but make sure that you return the wine/stock mixture back to the pan and continue to simmer. Chop mushrooms into bite–sized pieces.

2. Place olive oil in a heavy 5–quart saucepan or chef's pan. Add onion and sauté until onion starts to soften. Add rice, salt, and pepper and coat rice grains with olive oil mixture.

3. Add stock mixture 1 cup at a time and stir until each addition of liquid is absorbed. (This takes time and patience.) After last addition of stock is absorbed, add Parmigiano–Reggiano. When all of the stock is absorbed, which can take anywhere from 20–40 minutes, and rice grains are creamy, you can add the parsley and porcini.

VARIATIONS: ADD ANY OTHER COOKED INGREDIENTS, WHICH HAVE BEEN CUT INTO BITE–SIZE PIECES ALONG WITH THE PORCINI.

Cook's Tips

RISOTTO MUST BE SERVED IMMEDIATELY. IT DOES NOT WAIT!

Calories 315
Calories from Fat 65
Total Fat 7.0 g
Saturated Fat 2.1 g
Trans Fat 0.0 g
Cholesterol 5 mg
Sodium 335 mg
Potassium 280 mg
Total Carbohydrate 53 g
Dietary Fiber 4 g
Sugars 3 g
Protein 7 g
Phosphorus 180 mg

MEATLESS
MONDAYS

Stuffed Shells

1 pound jumbo pasta shells (about 40)

Nonstick cooking spray

12 ounces non-fat cottage cheese, small curd

15 ounces low-fat ricotta cheese

1 1/2 cups shredded reduced-fat 4 cheese Italian cheese mix (divided use)

1/2 cup grated fresh Parmigiano-Reggiano cheese

3 tablespoons chopped fresh Italian parsley

1/2 teaspoon fine sea salt

1/4 teaspoon freshly ground black pepper

10 ounces frozen chopped spinach, thawed and squeezed dry

6 cups Quick Marinara Sauce (see page 125)

This was one of my son's favorite dishes when he was growing up and I still enjoy making him a casserole of stuffed shells for "his night to cook."

SERVES 20 | SERVING SIZE 2 shells
EXCHANGES 1 1/2 Starch, 1 Vegetable, 1 Lean Meat, 1/2 Fat

1. Cook pasta according to package. Drain and set aside.

2. Preheat oven to 375°F. Spray two, 13 × 9–inch ovenproof dishes with nonstick cooking spray and set aside.

3. Place cottage cheese and ricotta in food processor or blender. Blend to smooth consistency. Transfer to large mixing bowl. Add 1 cup of Italian cheese, the Parmigiano–Reggiano, parsley, salt, pepper, and spinach. Mix well.

4. Fill each of the cooked shells with 1 tablespoon of the cheese filling. Place in casserole dishes, seam side up, in single layer. Spoon 1/2 of the Quick Marinara Sauce over each casserole. Top with the remaining cheese spread.

5. Cover and bake for 30 minutes until bubbly.

Cook's Tips

YOU CAN FREEZE THE UNBAKED CASSEROLE, BY COVERING THEM WITH PLASTIC WRAP AND THEN ALUMINUM FOIL.

TO REHEAT: DEFROST, REMOVE PLASTIC WRAP, REPLACE FOIL, AND PLACE IN 375°F OVEN FOR 30–45 MINUTES.

IF STILL FROZEN: REMOVE PLASTIC WRAP, REPLACE FOIL AND BAKE 60–75 MINUTES. IF BAKING DISH IS GLASS OR CERAMIC, PLACE IT IN A COLD OVEN SO THAT IT DOESN'T CRACK.

Calories 210
 Calories from Fat 55
Total Fat 6.0 g
 Saturated Fat 2.3 g
 Trans Fat 0.0 g
Cholesterol 15 mg
Sodium 510 mg
Potassium 445 mg
Total Carbohydrate 28 g
 Dietary Fiber 4 g
 Sugars 5 g
Protein 12 g
Phosphorus 225 mg

Tamale Casserole with Cheddar Crust

Nonstick cooking spray

FILLING

1 tablespoon extra virgin olive oil

1 medium green bell pepper, diced

1 medium onion, chopped

15 ounces canned pink beans, rinsed and drained well

15 ounces canned small white beans, rinsed and drained well

15 ounces canned chickpeas, rinsed and drained well

2 1/2 teaspoons ground cumin

1/4 teaspoon ground coriander

1/2 teaspoon dried oregano

1/2 teaspoon freshly ground pepper

28 ounces canned crushed tomatoes

1/2 cup medium-hot salsa

1/4 cup water

CRUST

1 1/2 cups yellow cornmeal

1 cup all-purpose flour

1 teaspoon baking powder

1/2 teaspoon baking soda

1/4 teaspoon salt

1 1/4 cups plain, low-fat yogurt

4 egg whites

2 tablespoons olive oil

1 cup shredded reduced-fat cheddar cheese (divided use)

1/2 cup chopped green onions

This dish is a crowd pleaser and a little bit different.

SERVES 12 | **SERVING SIZE** 1/12 recipe
EXCHANGES 2 1/2 Starch, 1 Vegetable, 1 Lean Meat, 1 Fat

1. Preheat oven to 375°F. Spray a 13 × 9 × 2-inch baking dish with cooking spray.

2. In a heavy nonstick skillet, heat oil over medium–high heat. Add the pepper and onion and sauté 6–8 minutes, or until the vegetables begin to soften. Add the beans and chickpeas. Toss well. Cook another 3 minutes for flavors to blend.

3. Stir in the cumin, coriander, oregano, and pepper and sauté, stirring for about 30 seconds. Add the tomatoes, salsa, and 1/4 cup water and bring to a boil. Remove from the heat and pour into prepared baking dish.

4. In a large bowl, mix together cornmeal, flour, baking powder, baking soda, and salt. Set aside.

5. In another large bowl, whisk together the yogurt, egg whites, and oil until well blended. Stir in 3/4 cup cheddar cheese and green onions. Pour the yogurt mixture over the cornmeal mixture and stir until blended. Spoon dollops of the mixture over the filling and spread evenly. Sprinkle with remaining 1/4 cup cheddar cheese.

6. Bake 25–30 minutes or until the filling is bubbly and the crust is lightly browned and firm. Cool a few minutes before serving.

Calories 305
  Calories from Fat 65
Total Fat 7.0 g
  Saturated Fat 2.1 g
  Trans Fat 0.0 g
Cholesterol 5 mg
Sodium 515 mg
Potassium 635 mg
Total Carbohydrate 48 g
  Dietary Fiber 9 g
  Sugars 8 g
Protein 14 g
Phosphorus 290 mg

Vegetable & Bean Chili

1 tablespoon canola oil

1 1/2 cups chopped Spanish onion (about 1 pound)

2 large green bell peppers, chopped

2 large carrots, sliced 1/2-inch thick

2 celery stalks, sliced 1/2 -inch thick

3 garlic cloves, minced

1 tablespoon minced jalapeño pepper (optional)

2 teaspoons dried oregano

1/8 teaspoon cayenne pepper

2 teaspoons ground cumin

Pinch ground cloves

2 (15-ounce) cans dark red kidney beans, drained and rinsed

4 cups canned no-salt-added peeled plum tomatoes (1 28-ounce can)

1/2 cup fresh chopped cilantro or flat Italian parsley

1/3 cup grated light cheddar cheese (for garnish)

1 bunch scallions, sliced (for garnish)

Chili is so full of flavor that you really don't need the meat.

SERVES 8 | SERVING SIZE 1 1/2 cups | EXCHANGES 1 Starch, 3 Vegetable, 1/2 Fat

1. Heat the oil in a large soup pot over medium–high heat. Add the onion, pepper, carrots, and celery and sauté until onion is translucent. Stir in the garlic, jalapeño, oregano, cayenne, cumin, and cloves. Sauté another 2–3 minutes.

2. Add the beans, tomatoes, and cilantro (or parsley) and bring to boil. Reduce the heat and simmer covered for 30-60 minutes or until flavors blend. Adjust seasonings before serving.

3. Ladle into bowls and garnish with cheese and sliced scallions.

Cook's Tips

WEAR RUBBER GLOVES WHEN SEEDING AND CHOPPING THE JALAPEÑO.

TOP WITH A DOLLOP OF PLAIN YOGURT OR COOKED POLENTA INSTEAD OF THE USUAL SOUR CREAM.

Calories 195
  Calories from Fat 30
Total Fat 3.5 g
  Saturated Fat 0.9 g
  Trans Fat 0.0 g
Cholesterol 0 mg
Sodium 475 mg
Potassium 945 mg
Total Carbohydrate 34 g
  Dietary Fiber 9 g
  Sugars 9 g
Protein 11 g
Phosphorus 200 mg

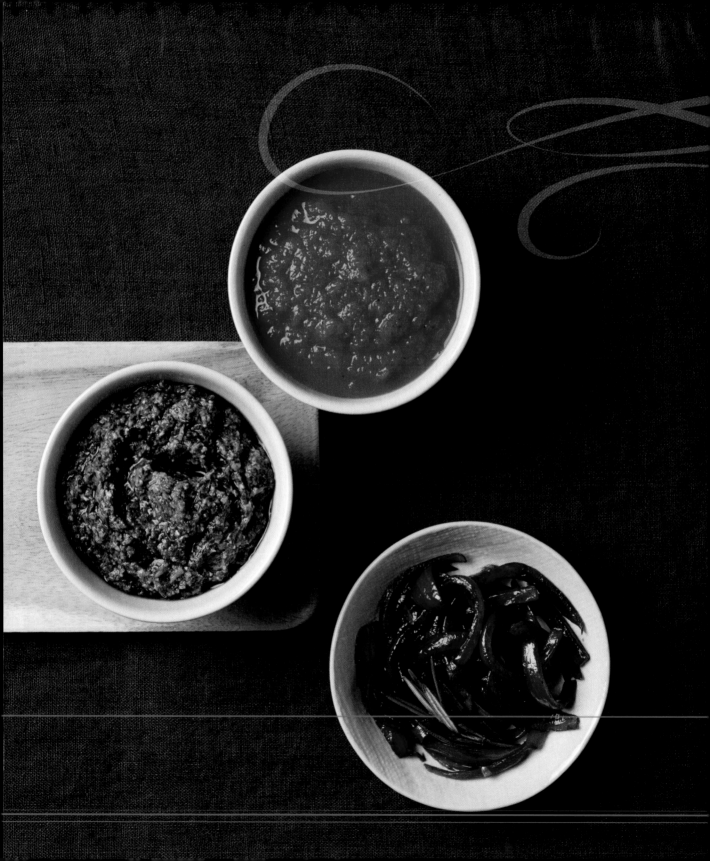

SPECIAL TOUCHES

Cinnamon Spiced Walnuts

1/4 cup sugar blend (I used
   Domino)

1 1/2 teaspoons ground cinnamon

1/4 teaspoon sea salt

1 egg white

2 cups walnuts

SERVES 16 | **SERVING SIZE** 2 tablespoons | **EXCHANGES** 2 Fat

1. Heat oven to 350°F. Combine sugar, cinnamon, and salt in a small bowl. Set aside. Beat egg white until foamy (soft peaks stage) in a medium bowl. Add spice mixture and blend well. Add walnuts and coat well.

2. Spread nuts on a parchment-lined baking sheet in a single layer. Bake 20–25 minutes, checking after 20 minutes. Cool slightly and break apart. Cool completely. These keep well for several weeks in an airtight container.

Calories 95
   Calories from Fat 70
Total Fat 8.0 g
   Saturated Fat 0.8 g
   Trans Fat 0.0 g
Cholesterol 0 mg
Sodium 40 mg
Potassium 60 mg
Total Carbohydrate 4 g
   Dietary Fiber 1 g
   Sugars 3 g
Protein 2 g
Phosphorus 45 mg

**SPECIAL
TOUCHES**

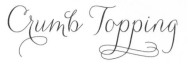

Crumb Topping

2 cups old-fashioned oats (not quick cooking)

1 cup Splenda Brown Sugar Blend

1 cup all-purpose flour

1/2 teaspoon salt

1 tablespoon cinnamon

1 cup walnut halves or pieces

4 ounces trans-fat–free margarine (such as Smart Balance)

This makes enough crumb topping to use on several pies, tarts, or batches of muffins. I like to prepare this and keep it in the freezer for a quick finishing touch on baked goods. It is also great when used as a topping for a sweet potato casserole.

SERVES 80 | **SERVING SIZE** 1 tablespoon | **EXCHANGES** 1/2 Carbohydrate

1. Place all ingredients in food processor fitted with steel blade. Process just until the butter is incorporated into the mixture. You will still have some large crumbs.

Calories 40
  Calories from Fat 20
Total Fat 2.0 g
  Saturated Fat 0.4 g
  Trans Fat 0.0 g
Cholesterol 0 mg
Sodium 25 mg
Potassium 20 mg
Total Carbohydrate 5 g
  Dietary Fiber 0 g
  Sugars 1 g
Protein 1 g
Phosphorus 15 mg

SPECIAL
TOUCHES

Caramelized Onions

2 tablespoons extra virgin olive oil

1 large (10 ounce) onion, about
1 1/2 cups, chopped

This little recipe can be used in many big ways—it is a great topping for Polenta Cheese Squares (page 110), a pizza, or bruschetta, and also a wonderful condiment for any grilled or roasted protein you are preparing, just to name a few options.

SERVES 12 | **SERVING SIZE** 1 tablespoon | **EXCHANGES** 1/2 Fat

1. Place extra virgin olive oil in 10-inch sauté pan. Add onion and cook on medium until onion becomes golden brown. Depending on your stove and pan, this can take different amounts of time. It should take at least 15 minutes and possibly up to 25 or 30 minutes.

Calories 30
Calories from Fat 20
Total Fat 2.5 g
Saturated Fat 0.3 g
Trans Fat 0.0 g
Cholesterol 0 mg
Sodium 0 mg
Potassium 30 mg
Total Carbohydrate 2 g
Dietary Fiber 0 g
Sugars 1 g
Protein 0 g
Phosphorus 5 mg

**SPECIAL
TOUCHES**

Garlic Crouton

Italian or French bread
Roasted Garlic (page 170)

1. Slice the bread on the diagonal and place on sheet pan. Place under broiler until crispy, approximately 3–5 minutes but watch it carefully.

2. Spread the roasted garlic on the grilled bread and use to garnish soups, salad, or stews.

Calories 45
  Calories from Fat 10
Total Fat 1.0 g
  Saturated Fat 0.2 g
  Trans Fat 0.0 g
Cholesterol 0 mg
Sodium 60 mg
Potassium 50 mg
Total Carbohydrate 7 g
  Dietary Fiber 1 g
  Sugars 1 g
Protein 2 g
Phosphorus 35 mg

SPECIAL
TOUCHES

Guacamole

2 avocados (about 1 pound or 1 cup mashed), purchased soft

1 lime, juiced

2 tablespoons chopped tomato

2 tablespoons finely minced or grated onion

1/8 teaspoon fine sea salt

Guacamole is one of those things that is very, very easy to make. It doesn't make sense to purchase something that is prepared and has added preservatives. This is great when served with the Enchilada Casserole (page 50), Mixed Bean Soup (page 57), with scrambled eggs, or with baked chips.

SERVES 10 | **SERVING SIZE** 2 tablespoons | **EXCHANGES** 1 Fat

1. Cut avocado in half and scoop flesh out with a spoon. Save pit. Place avocado in medium bowl and mash with fork. Add lime juice, tomato, onion, and salt. Blend well. Place avocado pit back in the guacamole and cover it tightly to help keep it from browning.

Cook's Tips

USE A BOX GRATER TO GRATE A SMALL ONION FOR FINELY MINCED ONION.

Calories 40
Calories from Fat 30
Total Fat 3.5 g
Saturated Fat 0.5 g
Trans Fat 0.0 g
Cholesterol 0 mg
Sodium 35 mg
Potassium 125 mg
Total Carbohydrate 3 g
Dietary Fiber 2 g
Sugars 0 g
Protein 1 g
Phosphorus 15 mg

SPECIAL TOUCHES

Mushroom Sherry Sauce

2 tablespoons extra virgin olive oil

1 shallot, minced (about 2 tablespoons)

10 ounces mushrooms, sliced

2 tablespoons flour

1/2 cup dry sherry

1/2–1 cup vegetable stock

1/2 cup Italian parsley, minced

This wonderful sauce is very versatile and can be used on anything! The type of stock can also be varied according to what you are serving this with.

SERVES 5 | SERVING SIZE 1/2 cup **| EXCHANGES** 1 Vegetable, 1 1/2 Fat

1. Place olive oil in sauté pan. Add shallots and mushrooms and cook until wilted. Add flour and cook 3 minutes.

2. Add sherry and stock and reduce sauce to desired consistency. Just before serving, add fresh parsley.

Calories 90
  Calories from Fat 55
Total Fat 6.0 g
  Saturated Fat 0.8 g
  Trans Fat 0.0 g
Cholesterol 0 mg
Sodium 100 mg
Potassium 285 mg
Total Carbohydrate 6 g
  Dietary Fiber 1 g
  Sugars 1 g
Protein 2 g
Phosphorus 70 mg

SPECIAL TOUCHES

Pesto

4 cloves garlic

1/2 cup pignoli (pine nuts)

4 cups fresh basil leaves, reserve 1 or more sprigs (for garnish)

3/4 cup freshly grated Parmigiano-Reggiano cheese

1/4 cup extra virgin olive oil

Pesto means paste in Italian. The original Genovese pesto was made using a mortar and pestle so the texture was not perfectly smooth. Be careful when using your food processor not to overmix. For a lower-fat or thinner version of pesto, you can replace some of the oil with chicken or vegetable stock.

SERVES 16 | **SERVING SIZE** 1 tablespoon | **EXCHANGES** 1 1/2 Fat

1. Place garlic and pignoli in food processor and process until minced. Add basil and Parmigiano-Reggiano cheese and process until smooth. Add olive oil and pulse until well blended.

Cook's Tips

PESTO DOES NOT HAVE TO BE PERFECTLY SMOOTH.

PESTO IS GREAT ON PASTA, IN SALAD DRESSING, ON BAKED POTATOES, OR SWIRLED INTO A SOUP OR RISOTTO.

VARIATIONS: BLACK OLIVE—ADD 1/2 CUP PITTED BLACK OLIVES; SUN-DRIED TOMATO—ADD 1 CUP REHYDRATED SUN-DRIED TOMATOES (NOT IN OIL); ARUGULA OR SPINACH—REPLACE SOME OF THE BASIL WITH ARUGULA OR SPINACH.

Calories 75
Calories from Fat 65
Total Fat 7.0 g
Saturated Fat 1.5 g
Trans Fat 0.0 g
Cholesterol 5 mg
Sodium 25 mg
Potassium 80 mg
Total Carbohydrate 1 g
Dietary Fiber 1 g
Sugars 0 g
Protein 2 g
Phosphorus 60 mg

SPECIAL TOUCHES

Porcini Mushroom Sauce for Pasta or Vegetables

1 1/2 tablespoons extra virgin olive oil

1/4 cup all-purpose flour

4 cups skim milk

1/4 cup dried porcini mushrooms, broken into small pieces

1/2 teaspoon fine sea salt

1/4 teaspoon ground black pepper

1/2 cup freshly chopped Italian parsley

This low-fat cream sauce with porcini mushrooms is delicious with pasta, steamed vegetables, or any grilled protein. It is versatile and freezes well.

SERVES 8 | SERVING SIZE 1/2 cup | EXCHANGES 1/2 Fat-Free Milk, 1/2 Fat

1. Place olive oil in large saucepan. Heat and add flour. Cook the flour 1–2 minutes until it just begins to turn brown. Slowly whisk in milk. Bring to boil and immediately turn to low. Add porcini. Cook until thickened. Taste and add salt, pepper, and parsley.

Calories 80
  Calories from Fat 20
Total Fat 2.5 g
  Saturated Fat 0.4 g
  Trans Fat 0.0 g
Cholesterol 0 mg
Sodium 200 mg
Potassium 220 mg
Total Carbohydrate 10 g
  Dietary Fiber 0 g
  Sugars 6 g
Protein 5 g
Phosphorus 130 mg

Roasted Garlic

4 large heads of garlic
2 teaspoons extra virgin olive oil
1/2 teaspoon fine sea salt

Roasted garlic is a great staple to have on hand. It adds depth of flavor to salad dressings, sauces, soups, stews, and makes a great spread for a crouton or sandwich. The flavor of garlic mellows as you go from fresh to sautéed to roasted.

SERVES 6 | **SERVING SIZE** 1 tablespoon | **EXCHANGES** 1 Vegetable

1. Preheat oven to 400°F.

2. Using chef's knife, slice a thin piece off the top or stem end of the garlic to expose most of the cloves. Place heads on large sheet of aluminum foil and drizzle with just enough olive oil to moisten the garlic, approximately 1/2 teaspoon per head. This will vary depending on the size of the garlic. Sprinkle each with a pinch of sea salt.

3. Wrap garlic up tightly and place in ceramic dish. Bake approximately 45 minutes or until very soft to the touch and a spreadable consistency. (Cooking time will vary depending on the freshness, size, and water content of the garlic.)

4. Squeeze the roasted garlic out of the husk. To make a spread, simply mash garlic and place in serving dish.

~**VARIATIONS:** BREAK CLOVES APART, DRIZZLE WITH OIL, SEASON WITH SALT AND PEPPER, AND ROAST IN 20–30 MINUTES;
PEEL GARLIC CLOVES, DRIZZLE WITH OIL, SEASON WITH SALT AND PEPPER, AND ROAST IN FOIL FOR 20 MINUTES.

Calories 30
  Calories from Fat 10
Total Fat 1.0 g
  Saturated Fat 0.2 g
  Trans Fat 0.0 g
Cholesterol 0 mg
Sodium 20 mg
Potassium 60 mg
Total Carbohydrate 5 g
  Dietary Fiber 0 g
  Sugars 0 g
Protein 1 g
Phosphorus 25 mg

SPECIAL TOUCHES

Roasted Red Pepper Coulis

4 red bell peppers

A coulis is simply a thick puree or sauce. This one makes a beautiful and tasty finishing touch for your dishes.

SERVES 8 | SERVING SIZE 1/4 cup | EXCHANGES 1 Vegetable

1. Place whole peppers directly on a grill or gas burner or under your broiler. Roast until they are completely blackened on the outside. Place in a bowl and cover tightly with plastic wrap for at least 15 minutes. Once cooled, you can peel away the blackened skin.

2. Place the roasted pepper in the food processor and purée until fine.

Calories 20
  Calories from Fat 0
Total Fat 0.0 g
  Saturated Fat 0.0 g
  Trans Fat 0.0 g
Cholesterol 0 mg
Sodium 0 mg
Potassium 155 mg
Total Carbohydrate 4 g
  Dietary Fiber 1 g
  Sugars 3 g
Protein 1 g
Phosphorus 20 mg

SPECIAL TOUCHES

Rosemary Balsamic Onions

1 tablespoon extra virgin olive oil

4 cups sliced onions, red and white combined (about 4 medium)

1/2 teaspoon Salt & Pepper Blend (page viii)

2 sprigs fresh rosemary (about 1 tablespoon)

2 tablespoons balsamic vinegar

1 tablespoon water

This is my version of a traditional Italian condimenti. It is great with a roast such as filet mignon or pork. It can also be made several days ahead.

SERVES 9 | **SERVING SIZE** 1/4 cup | **EXCHANGES** 1 Vegetable, 1/2 Fat

1. Place extra virgin olive oil in a large sauté pan. Add onions and Salt & Pepper Blend. Toss well. Sauté until onions begin to brown, about 10 minutes. Add rosemary and vinegar and turn off heat. If desired, add water to give a little more sauce.

Calories 45
Calories from Fat 15
Total Fat 1.5 g
Saturated Fat 0.2 g
Trans Fat 0.0 g
Cholesterol 0 mg
Sodium 90 mg
Potassium 105 mg
Total Carbohydrate 7 g
Dietary Fiber 1 g
Sugars 3 g
Protein 1 g
Phosphorus 20 mg

SPECIAL TOUCHES

Basic Vinaigrette

1/4 cup vinegar

Pinch fine sea salt

Freshly ground pepper, to taste

Fresh herbs such as chives or basil, chopped (optional)

1/2 cup extra virgin olive oil

This vinaigrette can be used as a salad dressing or as a marinade.

SERVES 12 | **SERVING SIZE** 1 tablespoon | **EXCHANGES** 2 Fat

1. Place vinegar, salt, pepper, and herbs, if desired, in medium mixing bowl. Start whisking and slowly stream in the olive oil. Taste after 1/2 cup has been added. The amount of oil required to balance the vinegar will depend on the vinegar selected.

~**VARIATIONS:** USE DIFFERENT TYPES AND FLAVORS OF VINEGAR; ADD 1–2 DROPS ORANGE OIL OR ORANGE EXTRACT; ADD CHOPPED, FRESH HERBS; ADD ROASTED GARLIC; FRESH RASPBERRIES; CRUSHED CRANBERRIES; MAKE A FRENCH VINAIGRETTE BY ADDING 1 TEASPOON DIJON MUSTARD.

Cook's Tips

SLOWLY WHISKING IN THE OIL ALLOWS FOR BETTER EMULSION.

Calories 80
  Calories from Fat 80
Total Fat 9.0 g
  Saturated Fat 1.2 g
  Trans Fat 0.0 g
Cholesterol 0 mg
Sodium 15 mg
Potassium 0 mg
Total Carbohydrate 0 g
  Dietary Fiber 0 g
  Sugars 0 g
Protein 0 g
Phosphorus 0 mg

SPECIAL
TOUCHES

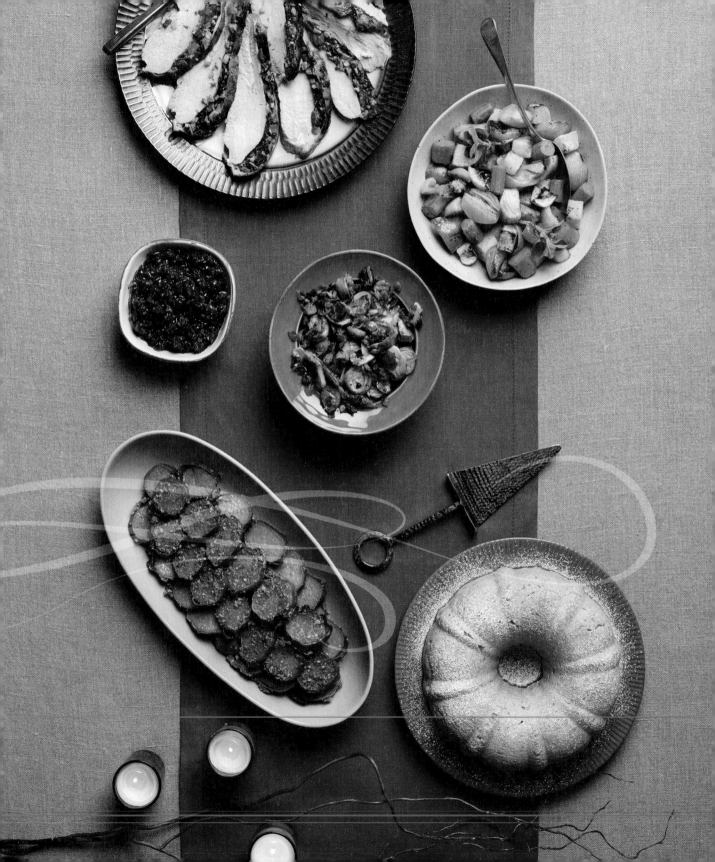

THANKSGIVING

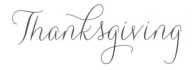

I love Thanksgiving. It is MY holiday, the time that I have the largest number of family members in one place for the longest time. Our family has a plan that works for us and even though we number 25ish, it is not too daunting.

Over the years, we have had various friends, in-laws, and co-workers who may have needed a place to go. Isn't that what Thanksgiving is all about? I am grateful for the fact that I have a table full of loved ones each year and am happy to share dinner with extended family and friends.

Thanksgiving is commonly referred to as the biggest meal of the year, so now is the time to start making your lists so dinner planning and preparation will be a breeze. I believe that only those people who enjoy cooking should take on Thanksgiving dinner.

My son refers to Thanksgiving as the nicest holiday of the season because we are not yet exhausted with shopping, wrapping, and other associated holiday chaos. I must agree with him (he's brilliant, you know). Your preparation can begin with the checklists provided here. Many of us have the same guest list every year; however, if your Thanksgiving seems to change from year to year, confirm guests as early as possible or commit to where you are going to have dinner so that you or your host(ess) can plan accordingly.

Let's talk turkey. The turkey is the Thanksgiving centerpiece and it's actually the easiest part of the meal. My readers and students frequently ask how to get everything to come out at the same time. The simplest answer to that question is to cook the turkey with plenty of time before serving so that the turkey can rest for 30–60 minutes. This gives you the time you need to reheat other food in your oven and put the final touches on things. A turkey will be moister and more flavorful if it is allowed to rest, meaning that the juices will be absorbed back into the meat rather than being released when you start slicing too soon after removing from the oven. So give yourself a little extra time by building a generous resting period into your plan before it's time to serve dinner.

The perfectly cooked turkey is rather simple. Here's all you need to do to have a perfectly prepared bird. Preheat the oven to 325°F. Remove turkey from bag. Remove giblet package from neck skin area. With legs facing away, press one leg down near leg clamp to release. Release other leg. Do not remove clamp from turkey. Remove neck from body cavity. Rinse inside and outside of turkey with cold water. Drain well and pat dry.

If stuffing turkey, allow 3/4 cup stuffing per pound of turkey. Bake any extra stuffing in a casserole dish. Stuff turkey just before roasting, not ahead, as this is unsafe. Re-tuck legs in clamp. Roast immediately. Place turkey in roaster or in shallow pan with rack. Brush turkey with extra virgin olive oil. Opening the oven door will slow cooking time, so using a meat thermometer is recommended. Insert thermometer into the thickest part of the breast without touching the bone. Thermometer should read 165°F when turkey is done. Start checking with a meat thermometer 1 hour before you expect the turkey to be done, allowing 15 minutes per pound.

When turkey is golden brown, cover with a loose tent of aluminum foil to prevent over browning. Alternative checks for doneness are: leg joint moves freely when the drumstick is rotated, or when a fork is inserted into the deepest part of the leg joint the juices are clear.

Remove turkey from pan to serving platter, reserving dripping in pan for gravy, if desired. Let turkey stand at least 10 to 15 minutes and up to one hour before carving, to allow juices near the surface of the skin to be redistributed for juicier meat and easier carving. A turkey can rest up to 1 hour and still be hot.

Make gravy during standing time and garnish turkey with fresh herb sprigs, if desired. Side dishes can be done ahead and frozen so that all you have to do is take them out of your freezer on Wednesday and reheat on Thursday while the turkey is resting.

THANKSGIVING CHECK LIST

- Clean out pantry, fridge, and freezer so that you can make room for holiday groceries.
- Do you have all your recipes selected so that you can make your shopping list? Place them in a folder so that they are at your fingertips when you need them.
- Do the mixer, blender, and food processor all work correctly—do you have the necessary attachments?
- Are your kitchen knives sharp?
- Inventory glassware, dishes, flatware, and serving pieces.
- Do you have enough seating? You will be surprised how large the number can be!
- Do you have enough linens?
- Do you want to purchase a new tablecloth?

- If you have a large group, should you make place cards? They alleviate the last-minute confusion at the table.
- Do you have enough candles?
- Which wine will you serve? Think not only about the turkey but the other dishes that have more deliberate flavors. There is a lot going on with both sweet and savory. Beaujolais or Pinot Noir are good choices. I am also considering a Rosé this year.
- Will there be overnight guests? Do you have enough bedding, towels, etc.
- What will your guests be bringing; pin them down to a specific category such as dessert or appetizer. Don't let the notoriously late bring appetizers.

PLAN THE MENU

- First course or hors d'oeuvres?
- Turkey—Decide what kind of turkey you will have, fresh, frozen, will it be given to you? If necessary, order your turkey from your local butcher or a farmers' market.
- Mashed or sweet potatoes, or both?
- Vegetables—fresh or frozen. Using some frozen can help lighten the workload.
- Dressing or stuffing?
- Bread or rolls?
- Cranberry sauce—will it be canned or do you make it yourself?
- Gravy or no gravy?
- Desserts—Make you own or have your guests bring them? (I suggest having your guests bring them.)
- Wine, sparkling water, or non-alcoholic beverages? (It's a good idea to have them all onhand.)

SHOPPING LIST

Begin purchasing staple items (pick up a few each time you go to the store for something else)

- Turkey or turkey breast
- Chicken, vegetable, mushroom, or turkey broth
- Potatoes—white or sweet, can these be made ahead and frozen?
- Onions, garlic, and fresh herbs
- Vegetables
- Fruit and nuts (make a great centerpiece and serves as a light dessert)
- Butter
- Extra virgin olive oil
- Nonstick cooking spray
- Fine sea salt
- Peppercorns for the peppermill
- Extra paper towels, toilet tissue, and guest towels
- Dishwashing soaps
- Pot scrubbies
- Plastic wraps
- Aluminum foil
- Foil pans to make cleanup easier and to fill with leftovers for guests to take home.
- Freezer bags in all sizes
- Parchment paper
- Turkey dog and cat food (if your guests are bringing their furry friends)

HOW TO COOK A TURKEY

Estimate the number of guests and allow 1–1 1/2 pounds per person. Plan on cooking your turkey approximately 15 minutes per pound. Use a meat thermometer to take the guesswork out of cooking times. The thermometer should read 170°F in the leg and thigh joint. Do not depend on the popup timer; it pops up at a higher temperature, so the turkey may be done before it pops up. Avoid overcooking with a $10 instant-read meat thermometer. Give the turkey the food equivalent of your aerobic cooldown and let it rest 20–60 minutes for easier slicing and juicier slices. This also gives you time to put finishing touches on side dishes and frees up the oven for other items as well.

There are many ways to prep your turkey for the oven. I prefer something very simple. I rub my turkey with extra virgin olive oil, salt, and pepper and stuff it with carrots, celery, and onions. Dried herbs can burn during the long cooking time. I put a couple of inches of white wine in the bottom of the roasting pan for basting. The juice from the turkey will give you more basting liquid.

Cooking two smaller turkeys, rather than one large one, might be more appropriate depending on your oven size and other demands on the oven. Make sure the turkey you purchase will fit in your oven and refrigerator. If you have a large crowd and need to cook two, cook one a day ahead, carve, cover, and reheat gently on the day of the gathering. The second turkey can be the bird everyone oohs and aahs over.

Remember to allow adequate defrosting time for frozen turkeys. You should figure 24 hours of defrosting in the refrigerator for every 5 pounds of turkey. This can take 3–5 days, not counting the day of cooking. If you are planning a fresh turkey, decide where you will purchase it and order it now.

You can also call the following turkey hotlines with turkey questions: The USDA at 888–674–6854, Butterball at 800–288–8372, or Reynolds Turkey Hotline at 800–745–4000.

Also, remember to store leftovers within 2 hours to avoid any food safety risks.

A FEW EXTRA TIPS

- Select music ahead of time. Set up the CD player early in the day or a day ahead.
- Use lots of candles for atmosphere. Group multiple candleholders as centerpieces.
- Get all serving pieces, ice buckets, trays, etc., out ahead of time and place sticky notes on them as to what menu item they will hold to avoid last-minute rummaging through cabinets. This will be beneficial to those helping you at the last minute.
- Prepare garnishes for drinks and plates a day before (i.e., slice lemons, wash herbs, etc.).
- Use recipes that can be made ahead of time.

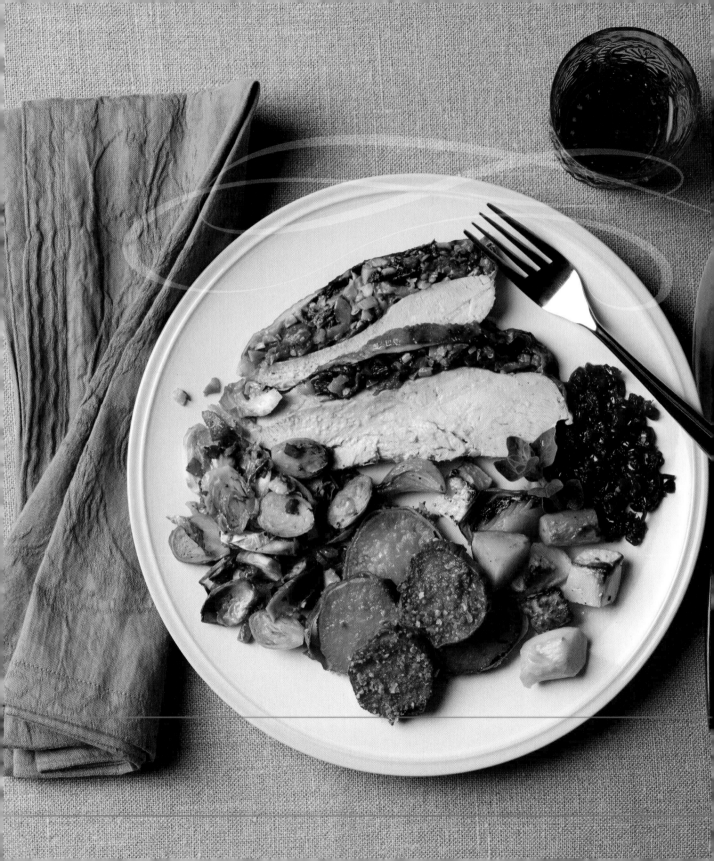

Baked Baby Pumpkins

1 baby pumpkin per guest (aka Jack Be Littles)

1 tablespoon shredded apple per pumpkin

1 teaspoon Crumb Topping (page 163)

Extra virgin olive oil for brushing on outside of pumpkins (you won't be eating the skin)

This dish is really fun to serve. Everyone gets his or her own little pumpkin. I like to serve it as an appetizer while people are arriving on Thanksgiving. It is also a wonderful side dish.

SERVES 1 | **SERVING SIZE** 1 pumpkin | **EXCHANGES** 1/2 Starch

1. Preheat oven to 400°F.

2. Scrub the pumpkins and place on a parchment-lined baking sheet. Brush very lightly with extra virgin olive oil.

3. Bake the pumpkins until you can insert a knife very easily.

4. Remove from oven and cool slightly. Cut the tops off. Remove seeds and discard.

5. Fill each pumpkin with apple and crumb topping. Return to oven and bake another 15 minutes or until bubbly.

Calories 30
  Calories from Fat 5
Total Fat 0.5 g
  Saturated Fat 0.1 g
  Trans Fat 0.0 g
Cholesterol 0 mg
Sodium 10 mg
Potassium 175 mg
Total Carbohydrate 6 g
  Dietary Fiber 1 g
  Sugars 2 g
Protein 1 g
Phosphorus 25 mg

Braised Brussels Sprouts with Pancetta

2 cups fresh Brussels sprouts

1 tablespoon extra virgin olive oil

2 garlic cloves, peeled and minced

2 shallots, thinly sliced

1 1/4 ounces finely chopped pancetta or turkey bacon

1/2–1 cup no-salt-added chicken or vegetable stock

1/4 teaspoon freshly ground pepper (optional)

1/4 teaspoon fine sea salt (optional)

Pancetta is Italian bacon that is rather low in fat. If you can't find pancetta try turkey bacon. Turkey bacon can vary in fat content by brand so be sure to read the label and find the brand lowest in fat.

SERVES 4 | SERVING SIZE 1/2 cup | **EXCHANGES** 1 Vegetable, 1 1/2 Fat

1. Trim the stem ends of the Brussels sprouts and remove outer leaves. Wash Brussels sprouts. Thinly slice the Brussels sprouts vertically (from stem end).

2. Place extra virgin olive oil in large sauté pan. Add garlic, shallots, pancetta, and Brussels sprouts. Cook 3–5 minutes until vegetables begin to soften and pancetta begins to brown. Add 1/2 cup stock and cook until tender. Add more stock as necessary. Season with salt and pepper, if desired.

Calories 95
Calories from Fat 55
Total Fat 6.0 g
Saturated Fat 1.5 g
Trans Fat 0.0 g
Cholesterol 5 mg
Sodium 340 mg
Potassium 265 mg
Total Carbohydrate 6 g
Dietary Fiber 2 g
Sugars 1 g
Protein 4 g
Phosphorus 85 mg

Herbed Bread Stuffing

2 tablespoons extra virgin olive oil

2 stalks celery, sliced

1 medium onion, diced

1 large apple, diced

1–2 teaspoons poultry seasoning, such as Bell's or McCormick

4 cups low-sodium chicken or vegetable stock

1 bag unseasoned stuffing cubes

1/2 cup fresh herbs, such as Italian parsley, thyme, sage, or chives, chopped (a combination of your favorite herbs will also work well)

SERVES 10 | **SERVING SIZE** 1/2 cup | **EXCHANGES** 2 Starch, 1/2 Fat

1. Place olive oil in large sauté pan. Add celery and onion and sauté until softened, approximately 3–5 minutes. Add apple and poultry seasoning. Toss well. Add stock and simmer 2–3 minutes. Add bread cubes and fresh herbs and toss well. Set aside to cool before stuffing poultry or pork.

2. You can also bake this stuffing in an ovenproof casserole rather than stuffing the bird. Bake at 350°F for 30 minutes. If you want crispy stuffing, you will bake uncovered. If you like a softer stuffing, you will want to cover.

VARIATIONS: USE 1 CUP DRIED FRUIT SUCH AS CRANBERRIES OR APRICOTS, SUN–DRIED TOMATOES, OR CHESTNUTS IN PLACE OF THE APPLE.

Calories 170
  Calories from Fat 40
Total Fat 4.5 g
  Saturated Fat 0.7 g
  Trans Fat 0.0 g
Cholesterol 0 mg
Sodium 280 mg
Potassium 215 mg
Total Carbohydrate 27 g
  Dietary Fiber 2 g
  Sugars 5 g
Protein 5 g
Phosphorus 65 mg

Cranberry Jalapeño Salsa

1–2 fresh jalapeño peppers

1 bag fresh cranberries, rinsed

1 small onion, cut in quarters and peeled

1 cup fresh cilantro, washed and torn into pieces that will fit in the food processor

3 tablespoons honey

1/2 teaspoon salt

This sweet, tart, hot salsa has been a hit every time I have served it. I love adding it to the Thanksgiving menu because of the cranberries. It is also great as a sauce for grilled chicken, fish, or pork.

SERVES 10 | SERVING SIZE 1/4 cup | EXCHANGES 1/2 Carbohydrate

1. Seed and roughly chop jalapeño. Wear gloves to avoid your hands getting hot.
2. Place all ingredients in food processor fitted with steel blade. Pulse until well blended. Can be made several days ahead and refrigerated.

Calories 35
  Calories from Fat 0
Total Fat 0.0 g
  Saturated Fat 0.0 g
  Trans Fat 0.0 g
Cholesterol 0 mg
Sodium 120 mg
Potassium 70 mg
Total Carbohydrate 9 g
  Dietary Fiber 2 g
  Sugars 5 g
Protein 0 g
Phosphorus 10 mg

Enlightened Herb Roast Chicken

5 pound roasting chicken

1/2 cup fresh basil leaves

1/4 cup fresh rosemary

1/2 cup fresh Italian parsley

5–6 fresh garlic cloves, sliced into rounds

1 teaspoon extra virgin olive oil

1/2 teaspoon fine sea salt

1/2 teaspoon freshly ground black pepper

This recipe would be a great alternative to a large turkey if you are having only two or four people on Thanksgiving or if your family is not fond of turkey. It is great when cooked on the grill.

SERVES 8 | SERVING SIZE 1/8 recipe | **EXCHANGES** 4 Lean Meat, 1/2 Fat

1. Clean chicken. Cut alongside breastbone separating the chicken into one big flat bird.

2. Remove basil, rosemary, and parsley from their stems. Mix with garlic slices.

3. Gently lift skin and tuck basil, rosemary, parsley, and garlic under skin.

4. Lightly brush the outside of the bird with olive oil (or use mister). Mix the salt and pepper together and rub on the outside of the bird.

5. Place skin side up on roasting pan lined with parchment and roast until golden and to an internal temperature of 165°F, as follows: Bake–400° for 1 hour, convection bake–375°F for 45 minutes, or grill on medium/low with lid closed–time will vary depending on grill.

~ **VARIATIONS:** SPLIT CORNISH HENS, WHICH WILL COOK IN 45 MINUTES; INDIVIDUAL CHICKEN PIECES, WHICH WILL ONLY TAKE 20–30 MINUTES TO COOK; FRESH OR PRESERVED LEMONS CAN BE USED IN ADDITION TO THE HERBS.

Calories 210
  Calories from Fat 70
Total Fat 8.0 g
  Saturated Fat 2.1 g
  Trans Fat 0.0 g
Cholesterol 90 mg
Sodium 160 mg
Potassium 290 mg
Total Carbohydrate 3 g
  Dietary Fiber 0 g
  Sugars 0 g
Protein 30 g
Phosphorus 210 mg

Garlic Mashed Potatoes

3 pounds Yukon gold potatoes,
   peeled and cut into 1-inch cubes

6 cloves garlic, peeled

1 teaspoon fine sea salt

4 cups chicken stock

Freshly ground pepper, to taste

These potatoes work very well as a do-ahead dish, which is very handy when you have so much to do on turkey day! They can be frozen in an ovenproof casserole dish, defrosted, and reheated in a 350°F oven until piping hot, approximately 45 minutes. Or prepare them up to 2 days ahead without the need to freeze.

SERVES 12 | **SERVING SIZE** 1/2 cup | **EXCHANGES** 1 starch

1. Place potatoes, garlic, salt, and pepper in heavy saucepan. Add stock and additional water to cover. Boil until potatoes are fork tender. Drain liquid from potatoes into a bowl and reserve to add back to potatoes.

2. Place potatoes in mixer bowl. Mix until smooth then add enough of the hot cooking liquid to achieve desired consistency.

Cook's Tips

YOU HAVE SAVED ALL THE VITAMINS AND MINERALS BY USING THE COOKING LIQUID! ALSO, BY USING THE COOKING WATER YOU WILL RETAIN THE POTATO STARCH, WHICH WILL ADD RICHNESS TO THE DISH.

YOU CAN ALSO USE VEGETABLE STOCK IN THIS DISH.

LEFTOVER COOKING LIQUID CAN BE USED IN SAUCES OR SOUPS.

POTATOES ARE ALSO GOOD WHEN USED AS DUCHESSE POTATOES, PIPED THRU A PASTRY BAG AND PUT ON TOP OF A POTPIE.

Calories 80
   Calories from Fat 0
Total Fat 0.0 g
   Saturated Fat 0.0 g
   Trans Fat 0.0 g
Cholesterol 0 mg
Sodium 125 mg
Potassium 325 mg
Total Carbohydrate 18 g
   Dietary Fiber 2 g
   Sugars 1 g
Protein 2 g
Phosphorus 45 mg

Golden Roasted Turkey Breast with Orange Zest, Spinach & Sun-Dried Tomato Stuffing

STUFFING

1 tablespoon extra virgin olive oil

1/2 cup finely chopped onion

1 cup plus 2 tablespoons no-salt-added chicken or vegetable stock (divided use)

2 cups chopped mushrooms

2 garlic cloves, finely minced

2 cups packed baby spinach leaves

2 tablespoons sun-dried tomatoes (not in oil), chopped

1 teaspoon grated orange zest

1/4 cup fresh basil

Freshly ground pepper

1–1 1/4 pounds boneless turkey breast with skin, aka turkey London broil

I often hear that people don't like to cook a whole turkey, so I am suggesting another delicious and beautiful option. This stuffing recipe can also double as a side dish or can be tossed with pasta for a quick meal.

SERVES 4 | SERVING SIZE 1/4 recipe | EXCHANGES 1 Vegetable, 3 Lean Meat

1. In sauté pan combine olive oil, onion, and stock. Cook, stirring over low heat, until onion is tender. This will take about 5 minutes.

2. Add the mushrooms and cook, stirring until tender and moisture has evaporated, approximately 3–5 minutes.

3. Add garlic and cook about 1 minute. Stir in spinach and cook, stirring until wilted, about 1 minute.

4. Add sun-dried tomatoes, orange zest, basil, and a grinding of fresh black pepper. Remove from heat. Cool.

5. Stuff mixture under the skin of turkey breast. Place in roasting pan and pour 1 cup additional stock or wine over turkey breast. Refrigerate until ready to roast.

6. Roast in a 375°F convection oven (25–30 minutes) or a 400°F standard oven (40–45 minutes) until internal temperature reaches 165°F. Can be basted with pan juices during roasting. Remove skin before serving.

Cook's Tips

SLICE LIKE A LONDON BROIL SO THAT YOU GET LAYERS OF TURKEY, STUFFING, AND GOLDEN BROWN SKIN.

Calories 180
Calories from Fat 55
Total Fat 6.0 g
Saturated Fat 1.3 g
Trans Fat 0.0 g
Cholesterol 50 mg
Sodium 255 mg
Potassium 660 mg
Total Carbohydrate 6 g
Dietary Fiber 2 g
Sugars 3 g
Protein 25 g
Phosphorus 230 mg

Pumpkin Soup Served in a Pumpkin

1 4–5 pound pumpkin

1 small onion, diced

1 tablespoon extra virgin olive oil

3 large carrots, thinly sliced

2 teaspoons no-added-salt tandoori seasoning

1 small potato, grated

16 ounces vegetable stock

Water

I like to use a hollowed-out pumpkin as a serving tureen at the table. If I am having a stand-up cocktail hour, I use tiny espresso cups.

SERVES 4 | **SERVING SIZE** 1/4 recipe | **EXCHANGES** 2 Starch

1. Preheat oven to 400°F.

2. Wash the pumpkin and place it on a baking sheet. Place the baking sheet in the oven and roast the pumpkin until a knife inserted near stem feels tender. This will take about an hour.

3. Cut the lid and remove seeds. Scoop out as much flesh as possible. Try not to damage the pumpkin so that you can use it as a serving bowl.

4. Place onion and oil in soup pot. Cook onions on medium until translucent. Add carrots, tandoori, and potato and cook until fork tender. Add pumpkin and stock. Purée with stick blender. Add water to desired consistency. Cook at least 20 minutes.

Calories 155
Calories from Fat 35
Total Fat 4.0 g
Saturated Fat 0.6 g
Trans Fat 0.0 g
Cholesterol 0 mg
Sodium 155 mg
Potassium 1080 mg
Total Carbohydrate 29 g
Dietary Fiber 6 g
Sugars 8 g
Protein 4 g
Phosphorus 135 mg

Roasted Butternut Squash Soup with Apple

1 (5-pound) butternut squash, cut into quarters

2 apples, peeled and quartered

6 cups vegetable or chicken stock

2 tablespoons finely minced ginger

1 cup evaporated skim milk, well shaken

1 teaspoon ground nutmeg

1/2 teaspoon ground cinnamon

Fine sea salt, to taste

Freshly ground black pepper, to taste

Better grocery stores sell the butternut squash already cut and seeded and this is a handy shortcut.

SERVES 12 | **SERVING SIZE** 1 cup | **EXCHANGES** 1 Starch

1. Preheat oven to 400°F. Roast squash on parchment–lined baking sheet until tender, approximately 20–30 minutes. Additionally, bake apples on parchment–lined baking sheet, approximately 15 minutes. Cool. Scrape flesh from squash and place in food processor with apples. Pulse until almost smooth.

2. Add stock and pulse again to make a smooth consistency. Place in large saucepan and add remaining ingredients. Bring to boil and reduce to simmer. Cook 20–30 minutes to allow flavors to blend.

3. Adjust seasonings before serving.

Cook's Tips

GARNISH WITH GARLIC CROUTON (PAGE 165), ROASTED RED PEPPER COULIS (PAGE 171), OR A DOLLOP OF NON–FAT SOUR CREAM OR LOW–FAT YOGURT, ALONG WITH SOME PUMPKIN, SQUASH, OR SUNFLOWER SEEDS.

CAN BE MADE A DAY OR TWO AHEAD.

GOOD SOURCE OF FIBER.

Calories 80
 Calories from Fat 0
Total Fat 0.0 g
 Saturated Fat 0.1 g
 Trans Fat 0.0 g
Cholesterol 0 mg
Sodium 100 mg
Potassium 480 mg
Total Carbohydrate 19 g
 Dietary Fiber 4 g
 Sugars 8 g
Protein 3 g
Phosphorus 115 mg

Roasted Root Vegetables With Garlic

1 large turnip (about 2 cups), scrubbed or peeled, cut into 1-inch chunks

3–4 carrots (about 1 cup), scrubbed or peeled, cut into 1-inch chunks

3–4 Yukon gold potatoes (about 2 cups), scrubbed, unpeeled, cut into 1-inch chunks

3–4 parsnips (about 1 cup), scrubbed or peeled, cut into 1-inch chunks

8–12 shallots (about 2 cups), peeled

1 tablespoon extra virgin olive oil

1 teaspoon fine sea salt

1 teaspoon freshly ground pepper

1 head garlic, cloves separated and peeled

Fresh herb sprigs (for garnish)

Drizzle of balsamic vinegar (optional)

I love serving roasted vegetables for any occasion, but root vegetables are especially nice for Thanksgiving. This dish can be prepared a day ahead. Once cooked and cooled, you can place them on an oven-safe platter, cover with aluminum foil, and refrigerate. On serving day, bring them to room temperature and reheat for about 20 minutes while the turkey is resting and being carved.

SERVES 9 | **SERVING SIZE** 2/3 cup | **EXCHANGES** 1 Starch, 2 Vegetable

1. Preheat oven to 425°F.

2. Place all prepped veggies in large bowl. Toss with olive oil, salt, and pepper. You will use less oil by tossing them in the bowl as opposed to drizzling on the baking sheet.

3. Line baking sheet with parchment. You might need more than 1 baking sheet. Place cut vegetables and garlic on baking sheet in single layer.

4. Roast to desired doneness, approximately 40–45 minutes Garnish with fresh herbs and drizzle of balsamic vinegar, if desired.

Calories 120
Calories from Fat 20
Total Fat 2.0 g
Saturated Fat 0.3 g
Trans Fat 0.0 g
Cholesterol 0 mg
Sodium 300 mg
Potassium 585 mg
Total Carbohydrate 25 g
Dietary Fiber 4 g
Sugars 4 g
Protein 3 g
Phosphorus 90 mg

Spaghetti Squash With Extra Virgin Olive Oil, Garlic & Parmigiano-Reggiano

1 spaghetti squash

2 tablespoons extra virgin olive oil

1 teaspoon granulated garlic powder

1/4 cup freshly grated Parmigiano-Reggiano cheese

SERVES 5 | **SERVING SIZE** 1 cup | **EXCHANGES** 2 Vegetable, 1 Fat

1. Wash spaghetti squash, pierce with a fork in several places, and place in microwave on high until skin is soft. This can take up to 30 minutes, but begin checking after 15 minutes. Let cool.

2. Cut squash in half and make "spaghetti." Using a fork, pull out individual strands of "spaghetti." Toss spaghetti squash with extra virgin olive oil, garlic powder, and Parmigiano-Reggiano.

VARIATIONS: YOU CAN ALSO TOP YOUR SPAGHETTI SQUASH WITH MARINARA, SAUTÉED MUSHROOMS, OR CHOPPED TOMATOES AND BASIL.

Calories 105
  Calories from Fat 65
Total Fat 7.0 g
  Saturated Fat 1.7 g
  Trans Fat 0.0 g
Cholesterol 5 mg
Sodium 55 mg
Potassium 190 mg
Total Carbohydrate 10 g
  Dietary Fiber 2 g
  Sugars 4 g
Protein 2 g
Phosphorus 50 mg

Spaghetti Squash With Quick Marinara Sauce

1 spaghetti squash
2 cups Quick Marinara Sauce (page 125)

Spaghetti squash is a great way to cut down on complex carbs.

SERVES 6 | **SERVING SIZE** 1 cup | **EXCHANGES** 3 Vegetable, 1/2 Fat

1. Wash spaghetti squash, pierce with a fork in several places, and place in microwave on high until skin is soft. This can take up to 30 minutes, but begin checking after 15 minutes. Let cool.

2. Cut squash in half and make "spaghetti." Using a fork, pull out individual strands of "spaghetti.

3. Top with Quick Marinara Sauce (page 125).

Calories 85
  Calories from Fat 25
Total Fat 3.0 g
  Saturated Fat 0.4 g
  Trans Fat 0.0 g
Cholesterol 0 mg
Sodium 325 mg
Potassium 495 mg
Total Carbohydrate 15 g
  Dietary Fiber 4 g
  Sugars 7 g
Protein 2 g
Phosphorus 55 mg

Sweet Potato & Chickpea Dip

1 pound sweet potato

2 cups canned chickpeas or white beans, drained and rinsed well

2 lemons, juiced

1 teaspoon cumin

1 garlic clove, peeled

1 tablespoon extra virgin olive oil

1/2 teaspoon fine sea salt

1/2 teaspoon ground black pepper

1/4 cup chopped Italian parsley

This dip is similar to hummus, but I left out the tahini (sesame paste), which is almost all fat and can be costly and not readily available. The sweet potato adds great nutritional value and flavor. It also has a bright fresh flavor with the added lemon.

SERVES 10 | **SERVING SIZE** 1/4 cup | **EXCHANGES** 1 Starch, 1/2 Fat

1. Peel sweet potato, cut into 1–inch cubes, and boil until fork tender. Drain well.

2. Place in food processor. Add remaining ingredients, except parsley. Pulse until smooth. Remove from food processor and stir in parsley. This recipe can be prepared up to two days ahead.

Cook's Tips

SUITABLE AS A DIP FOR PITA CHIPS AND RAW VEGETABLES OR AS A SPREAD FOR GRILLED VEGETABLE SANDWICHES.

Calories 100
  Calories from Fat 20
Total Fat 2.5 g
  Saturated Fat 0.3 g
  Trans Fat 0.0 g
Cholesterol 0 mg
Sodium 185 mg
Potassium 205 mg
Total Carbohydrate 17 g
  Dietary Fiber 3 g
  Sugars 4 g
Protein 3 g
Phosphorus 70 mg

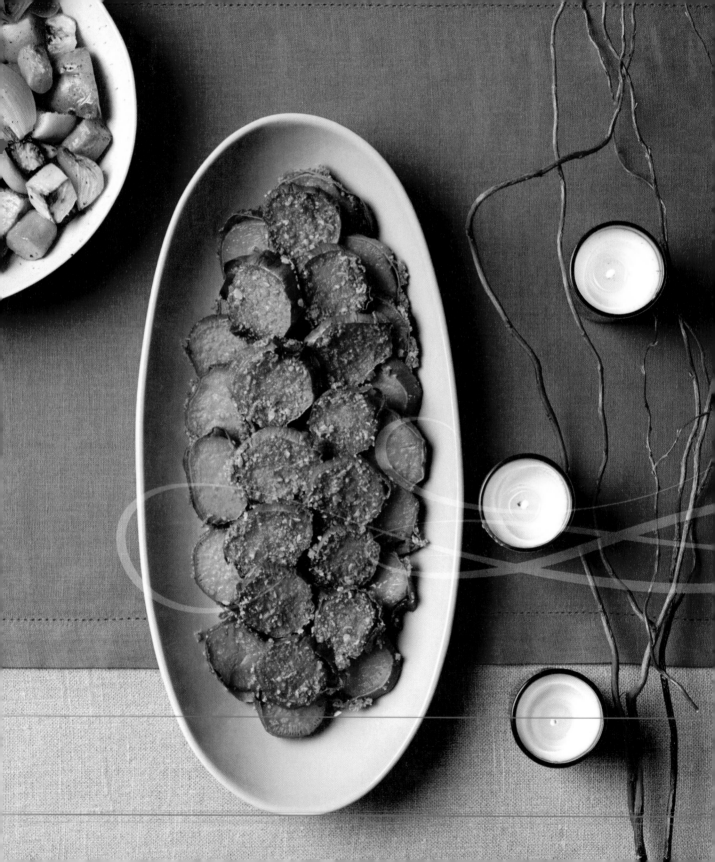

Sweet Potatoes With Crumb Topping

6 large sweet potatoes, baked until fork tender

1 cup Crump Topping (page 163)

I have never been a fan of the marshmallow–topped or the syrupy candied versions of sweet potato dishes. Those are all calorie laden, which made me want to create this recipe.

SERVES 12 | **SERVING SIZE** 1/12 recipe | **EXCHANGES** 2 Starch

1. Scrub the potatœs and bake at 375°F for an hour or so. The time will depend on the size of the potatoes.

2. Cool and slice 1/4 inch thick. Lay in a casserole dish and top with 1 cup Crumb Topping.

3. Bake for 30 minutes at 375°F.

Calories 135
  Calories from Fat 25
Total Fat 3.0 g
  Saturated Fat 0.5 g
  Trans Fat 0.0 g
Cholesterol 0 mg
Sodium 65 mg
Potassium 465 mg
Total Carbohydrate 26 g
  Dietary Fiber 4 g
  Sugars 7 g
Protein 3 g
Phosphorus 70 mg

THANKSGIVING

Thanksgiving Leftover Pot Pie

1 teaspoon extra virgin olive oil

1/2 cup chopped onion

1 clove garlic, minced

1 cup sliced celery

1 cup carrot, sliced 1/4 inch thick

2 tablespoons trans-fat-free tub margarine

1/4 cup all-purpose flour

2 cups no-salt-added chicken or turkey stock, plus additional, as needed

3 cups leftover turkey

1 cup frozen baby peas

2 tablespoons chopped Italian parsley

Fine sea salt, to taste

Freshly ground pepper, to taste

2 cups Garlic Mashed Potatoes (page 186)

This pot pie is a great way to use Thanksgiving leftovers. Most of the work is done for you. If you have leftover vegetables you can use them in place of the celery, onions, carrots, and peas in this recipe. Just assemble and bake. You can even freeze for later if you like.

SERVES 8 | SERVING SIZE 1/8 recipe | EXCHANGES 1 Starch, 2 Lean Meat, 1/2 Fat

1. Preheat oven to 375°F.

2. Heat olive oil to thinly film the bottom of the saucepan. Add onion and garlic and cook 2–3 minutes until onion begins to soften. Add celery and carrot and cook 5 minutes to soften. Set aside.

1. Melt margarine in a saucepan. Whisk in flour and mix well. Mixture will be dry. Gradually add 1 cup stock to saucepan. Cook 2–3 minutes until mixture begins to thicken and takes on a golden color. Add turkey, peas, parsley, and additional stock to achieve desired consistency (some like it soupy, some like it thicker). Add salt and pepper to taste.

1. Place mixture in baking dish and top with mashed potatoes. Bake at 375°F for approximately 25 minutes or until golden.

Cook's Tips

FLOUR MIXTURE MUST BE COOKED AT LEAST 2–3 MINUTES TO LOSE THE UNCOOKED FLOUR TASTE.

Calories 200
  Calories from Fat 55
Total Fat 6.0 g
  Saturated Fat 1.6 g
  Trans Fat 0.0 g
Cholesterol 40 mg
Sodium 190 mg
Potassium 500 mg
Total Carbohydrate 17 g
  Dietary Fiber 3 g
  Sugars 3 g
Protein 19 g
Phosphorus 175 mg

Turkey Breast Stuffed with Wild Rice, Fruit, and Herbs

WILD RICE STUFFING

1 cup wild rice

3 tablespoons minced shallots

1 bay leaf

1/4 teaspoon fine sea salt

3 cups no-salt-added chicken stock

1/2 cup chopped mixed fresh herbs, such as thyme, Italian parsley, chives, rosemary, or sage

1 cup chopped dried fruit, such as apricots and cherries

1 cup chopped nuts, such as walnuts or pecans

Freshly ground pepper

TURKEY

1 1/2 pounds boneless turkey breast with skin

2 teaspoons Salt & Pepper Blend (page viii)

Here is yet another alternative to cooking a large turkey. This also makes a lovely dinner party entrée. Prepare wild rice a day ahead or several hours in advance for quick preparation on the day you serve this special dish.

SERVES 6 | SERVING SIZE 1/6 recipe
EXCHANGES 1 Starch, 1 Fruit, 1 Vegetable, 4 Lean Meat, 1 1/2 Fat

1. Rinse rice under running water and pick out any grains that do not look good to you. Place rice, shallots, bay leaf, salt, and stock in a 4–quart pan and cook until rice is tender, approximately 45 minutes. Remove bay leaf. Add herbs, dried fruit, nuts, and pepper. Set aside to cool before stuffing turkey breast.

2. Preheat oven to 400°F. Place turkey breast on cutting board and butterfly. Pound to even thickness. Season with Salt & Pepper Blend.

3. Place stuffing over turkey breast and roll turkey breast to enclose. Tie at 3–inch intervals. Place on roasting rack and roast for approximately 45–60 minutes or until meat thermometer reads 155–160°F. Let rest at least 15 minutes before slicing. Remove skin before eating.

Cook's Tips

TO BUTTERFLY TURKEY BREAST: LAY THE BREAST ON A CUTTING BOARD AND SLICE THROUGH THE THICKEST PART OF THE BREAST SO THAT YOU END UP WITH A SPLIT BREAST THAT IS STILL CONNECTED IN THE MIDDLE. THE SURFACE AREA OF THE BUTTERFLIED BREAST WILL BE DOUBLE THE SIZE AND THINNER THAN THE ORIGINAL BREAST.

STUFFING CAN BE USED WITH CHICKEN, TURKEY, OR PORK AND CAN BE MADE A DAY AHEAD.

Calories 415
  Calories from Fat 135
Total Fat 15.0 g
  Saturated Fat 1.5 g
  Trans Fat 0.0 g
Cholesterol 75 mg
Sodium 215 mg
Potassium 730 mg
Total Carbohydrate 37 g
  Dietary Fiber 5 g
  Sugars 17 g
Protein 35 g
Phosphorus 425 mg

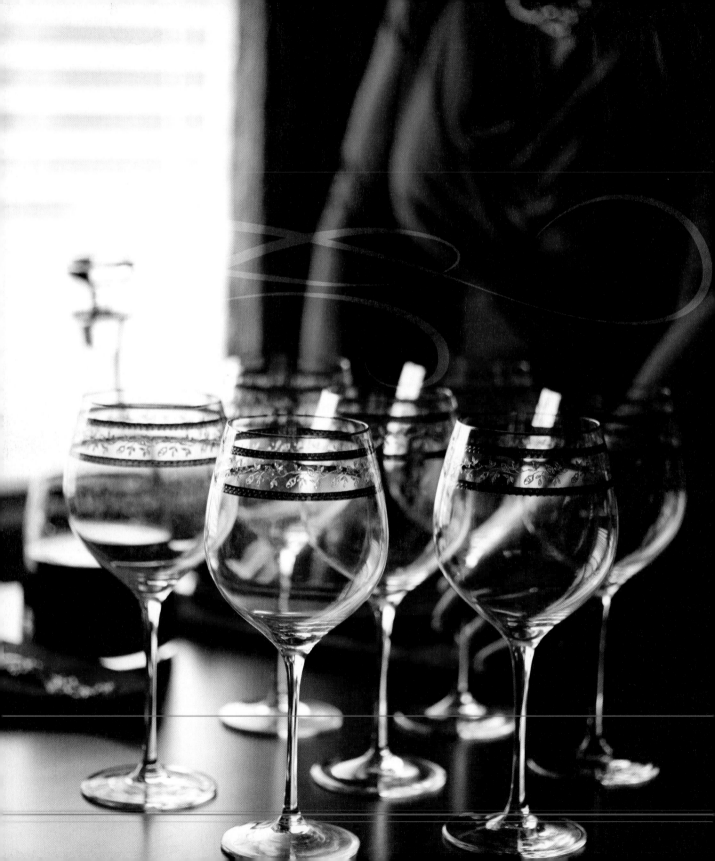

INDEX

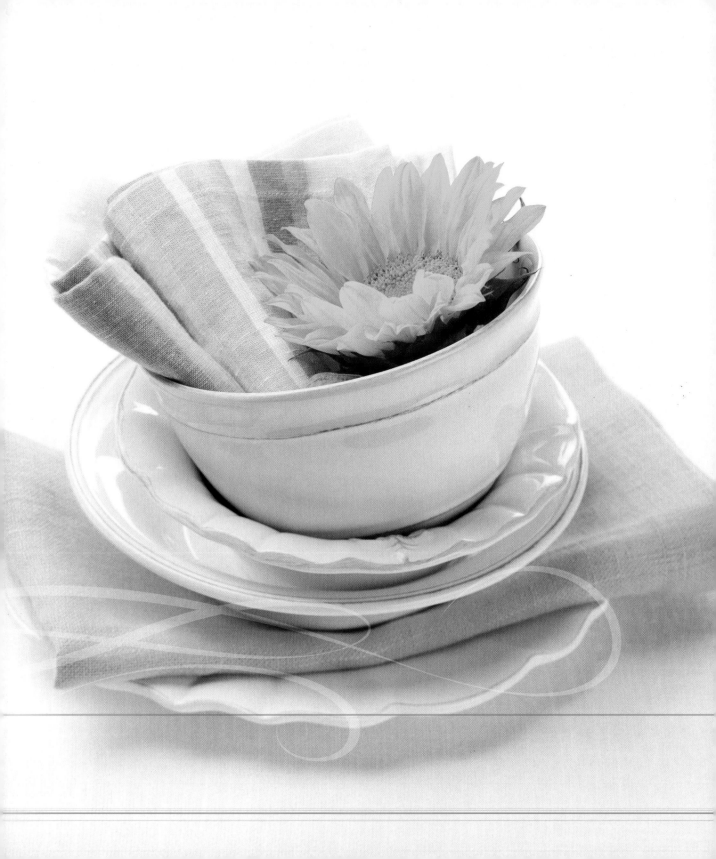

Subject Index

Note: Page numbers in **bold** refer to photographs.